THE BATTLE
FOR AMERICA'S SOUL

*Healthcare, the Culture War,
and the Future of Freedom*

C. L. Gray, MD

Copyright 2011 © by C. L. Gray

ISBN: 978-0-578-08054-3

Eventide Publishing
1126 10th St. Ln. NW
Hickory, NC 28601
(828) 256-9080
clgray@charter.net

Printed in the United States of America.

It could be said of me that in this book I have only made up a bunch of other men's flowers, providing of my own only the string that ties them together.

Michel de Montaigne (1533-1592)

"This book is dedicated to the thousands of patients I have cared for over the years and to the art of Hippocratic medicine."

Contents

PROLOGUE

Our world has changed. Even now, an unseen force grinds away, reshaping the nation Americans know and love. But reshaping her into what? This is the question.

A hidden hand seeks to remake this beloved country. Walking through an airport one can sense it. Conversations with friends and family reveal an inner turmoil, a mental pacing, a silent restlessness that lies just beyond view. Lines of unspoken apprehension flicker through a neighbor's face. Yes, the margin is gone, bank accounts leaner, and paychecks less certain... yet there is more. A fundamental transformation of culture marches forward. *We the People* see our future fading before us—this is the specter that haunts our dreams.

For perhaps the first time in American history, *We the People* fear our government. Not in a partisan sense, but in the sense that Washington seems deaf to the ordinary citizen, in the sense that politicians have squandered our children's future for the sake of political gain, in the sense the "greater good" now consumes individual liberty. Most of the world knows this fear. History is replete with examples of the ruling class holding the common citizen in contempt. But for the American, this is new. America's Founding Fathers built this constitutional republic on the concept of citizen statesmen stepping forward to lead under the rule of law... and then leave office to live once again as one of the governed. As Abraham Lincoln so eloquently observed, ours is a government *of the people, by the people, and for the people.*

Americans grow weary under the heavy hand of government, even as individual liberties slip away. As Washington burdens us with endless

7

regulation and overwhelming debt, *We the People* wonder if escape is possible, if we have reached the point of no return.

In January 2009, America embraced the bold new future of hope and change, trusting government to solve our nation's many problems—yet freedom may be the price we pay. Moved by a desire for social justice, Americans contemplated the socialism of Europe with enamored eye. In many quarters, cheers and accolades greeted the thought of government ensuring the healthcare of every American. However, liberty can be lost amidst the applause of men.

In these times of testing, history demands that America remember the best of who she is. Her Founding Fathers believed government derived its just power from the consent of the governed. *It is here she finds hope, for it is here that We the People find a Truth stronger than the political power of Washington. We the People* must remember our birthright and choose to act; *We the People* must reclaim our just position as the source of power in Washington. The notion that the ordinary citizen derives liberty from the good will of government would make the Founding Fathers spin in their graves.

> *Our Founding Fathers believed government derived its just power from the consent of the governed. It is here we find hope, for it is here that We the People find a Truth stronger than the political power of Washington.*

Americans must understand how they arrived in a place such as this. They must understand the forces that work to subjugate *We the People* to the strong arm of government. If liberty is to survive, we must lay down our political swords and remember our past. This is not a matter of Democrat vs. Republican; this is a matter of *We the People* vs. our government.

The task of restoring our nation's founding principles is profoundly difficult. A force that insidiously seeks this nation's destruction lies deeper than the partisan politics that consumes our nation's capitol. Two diametrically opposed worldviews battle for the soul of America. One seeks to dismantle the founding documents and transfer power to Washington; the other seeks to reinstate the wisdom of the Founding Fathers and return power to *We the People.* Because those who subscribe to each of these opposing worldviews believe their efforts are for the good of the nation, the resulting culture war pits American against American. Roman history warns that the danger to a great society lies within. *The only force strong enough to bring America to her knees is internal division. Ours is the peril of a nation divided—a land at war against herself.*

The Battle for America's Soul explores how America's culture war is reshaping the future of *We the People*. Even more, this book explains why this battle of worldviews threatens to wash away the cornerstones of this great nation, including the foundations of freedom. Americans enjoy the greatest freedoms on earth, but this privilege will be lost if *We the People* forget the universal Truths which preserve our liberty.

C. L. Gray, MD

CHAPTER ONE

LIBERTY LOST

When the people fear their government, there is tyranny;
when the government fears the people, there is liberty.
Thomas Jefferson (1743-1826)

"I'm not ready, I'm not ready to die. I've got things I'd still like to do."[1] Sixty-four-year-old Barbara Wagner wiped her tears as she spoke of her cancer's return.

After two years in remission Barbara's non-small cell lung cancer reappeared during the spring of 2008. Her oncologist recommended aggressive treatment with Tarceva, a new chemotherapy, but Oregon's state run health plan denied the potentially life altering drug. Instead, the State plan offered to pay for either hospice care or physician-assisted suicide.

In stunned disbelief Americans ask, "How can this be? Yes, this happens in Europe. I've heard stories of Britain's National Health Service delaying intervention until the patient dies or reports of physician-assisted suicide in the Netherlands. But in America?"

The answer is simple. Oregon state officials controlled the healthcare decision-making—not Barbara and her physician. Chemotherapy would cost the state $4,000 every month she remained alive; the drugs for physician-assisted suicide held a one-time expense of less than $100. Barbara's treatment plan boiled down to accounting. To cover chemotherapy state policy demanded a five percent patient survival rate at five years. As a new drug,

Tarceva did not meet this dispassionate criterion. To Oregon, Barbara was no longer a patient; she had become a "negative economic unit."

In 1994 Barbara's state established the Oregon Health Plan to give its working poor access to basic healthcare while limiting costs by "prioritizing care." In 1997 Oregon legalized physician-assisted suicide to offer "death with dignity" to patients who chose to die without further medical treatment. In the end, the State secured the power to ration healthcare in order to control its financial risk, even if that meant replacing a patient's chance to live with the choice of how to die.

> In the end, the State secured the power to ration healthcare in order to control its financial risk, even if that meant replacing a patient's chance to live with the choice of how to die.

When queried about withholding Barbara's treatment, Dr. Walter Shaffer, a spokesman for Oregon's Division of Medical Assistance Programs, explained the policy this way, "We can't cover everything for everyone. Taxpayer dollars are limited for publicly funded programs. We try to come up with policies that provide the most good for the most people."[2]

Dr. Som Saha, chairman of the commission that sets policy for the Oregon Health Plan, echoed Shaffer, "If we invest thousands and thousands of dollars in one person's days to weeks, we are taking away those dollars from someone [else]."[3]

Twice Barbara appealed the ruling. Twice Oregon denied her treatment.

The shortcomings of America's healthcare system confront both patient and physician daily. The myriad and complex questions that surround healthcare offer no easy answers. Yet, as Americans contemplate the future of healthcare, they must begin with this foundational question, *"Who should control the personal and complex process of medical decision-making? The patient together with his or her physician? Or the State?"*

Many politicians trumpet "universal healthcare" with emotive plea. "America is the only developed nation whose government does not provide healthcare for its citizens. We should be ashamed!" Yet behind the soaring rhetoric lies this sober truth: *Whoever pays holds the power to choose and the government cannot provide everything for everyone.* When the State controls the allocation of healthcare dollars, patients are left with no recourse. Both patient and physician are stripped of their autonomy.

Barbara now understood. When interviewed about the experience she reflected, "To say to someone, 'we'll pay for you to die, but not pay for you to live,' it's cruel. I get angry. Who do they think they are?"[4] The once unthinkable, State-sponsored euthanasia, circled Barbara with unflinching stare.

"We want every American to have access to healthcare." Who argues with this sentiment? Government compassion sounds so noble when first introduced. In fact, this well-intentioned motive fueled the creation of the State-sponsored health plan that denied Barbara chemotherapy. Even more, this same argument fueled much of the passion behind the federal Patient Protection and Affordable Care Act (PPACA) of 2010.

However, as *We the People* become more and more reliant on the government, inch by precious inch, our liberty slips away—we become powerless in dependency. For seniors, nothing drives this point home more than the PPACA. Washington cut $500 billion from Medicare simply to say, "we reduced the deficit." As President Ford once noted, "A government big enough to give you everything you want is a government big enough to take from you everything you have."[5]

Seduced by sweet words of compassion, the financial welfare of the State silently usurps the wellbeing of the individual citizen. Secure in the belief that government will care for its citizens, Americans slumber in complacency until one day, when needed most, *We the People* will awake to find liberty lost.

How did this happen? How did America reach a point in her history where a government "of the people, by the people, and for the people" can offer physician-assisted suicide rather than the hope of life? In search for the answer, recent history demonstrates that Barbara Wagner's experience with the Oregon Health Plan was not the first time individual liberty was subjected to the welfare of the State. Three years earlier the dread shadow of socialism had swept cold across our land. However, rather than seizing control of healthcare, the gaunt fingers of government reached to grasp private property. Americans must understand the link between these two sentinel events if they are to recognize the single greatest threat to American liberty today.

Whoever pays holds the power to choose and the government cannot provide everything for everyone.

Your Home is Not Your Own

Susette Kelo finally saved enough money to purchase a serene, though neglected, Victorian cottage. Her mind's eye played with the prospect of possibility. She gazed at her beleaguered little house, past the tangles of brush and overgrown grass, and envisioned a heartwarming home of simple charm. With energy drawn from every American's dream, Susette toiled to renovate the property. Dressed in a fresh coat of salmon-pink paint, her home overlooked a beautiful view of Long Island Sound. However, even as Susette basked in the comfort of her cozy abode, the city of New London, Connecticut quietly laid other plans.

Facing budget shortfalls during the 1990's, the city embarked on a redevelopment project to attract industry, jobs, and money. They needed land. On the day before Thanksgiving, 2000, the sheriff taped a letter to Susette's door condemning her newly restored home along with six other nearby properties. New London ordered Susette to vacate by the following March. The city intended to seize her new home.

Pfizer, one of the world's largest pharmaceutical companies, planned to build a 400,000 square foot, twenty-four acre research and development complex not far from Susette's home on the old New London Mills site. The city of New London hoped to capitalize on this infusion of cash by redeveloping ninety acres of neighboring waterfront property. Unfortunately Susette's house sat on this prime real estate. The prospect of increased tax revenue from the new houses, modern office space, new retail stores, and a luxury hotel proved impossible to resist. Clearly, New London would benefit by acquiring Susette's house and the surrounding land. If the city officials gained control of her property, they could then sell it to professional developers. Everyone was thrilled; everyone except Susette.

For five years Susette fought New London's seizure of her property. The city did not intend to exercise its Constitutional right of eminent domain for a *public use* ("public use" are the actual words of the Fifth Amendment—traditionally understood to be activities such as building public structures: schools, highways, railroads, military bases...). In this case, New London planned to resell Susette's property to *another private citizen* for the sole purpose of increasing the city's revenue.

The question before the Supreme Court was simple: Did a local government's economic benefit of redevelopment supersede Susette's right to live in the house she owned and renovated?

Robed in black, five Supreme Court Justices rocked the nation on June 23, 2005. With a stroke of a pen, *Kelo v. New London* declared the Fifth Amendment words "public use" really meant "public benefit." For the first time in United States history, local governments could seize newly renovated property from an American citizen and give it to a private developer purely for the welfare of government. If the transfer of property increased local tax revenue, it was considered "public benefit." American jurisprudence now considered this "settled law."

When Justices Ruth Bader Ginsberg, Stephen Breyer, John Paul Stevens, David Souter, and Anthony Kennedy loosed themselves from the actual words and original intent of the Fifth Amendment, tremors of a massive change in our understanding of the Constitution reverberated across the country. For these Justices, the Constitution's meaning was no longer fixed; the concept of original intent was outmoded, a relic of the past. The Constitution had become a "living, breathing document" whose meaning evolved with culture. These five Justices claimed sovereign power to determine what this new meaning should be. Rather than seeking to discern the original intent of the law and apply it to a given case, they expanded their Constitution role to "do good." However, whose good did they seek?

> For the first time in United States history, local governments could seize newly renovated property from an American citizen and give it to a private developer purely for the welfare of government.

The four remaining Justices (William Rehnquist, Antonin Scalia, Clarence Thomas, and Sandra Day O'Connor) opposed with stinging dissent. Clarence Thomas wrote:

> At the time of the founding, dictionaries primarily defined the noun "use" as "[t]he act of employing any thing to any purpose." The term "use," moreover, "is from the Latin *utor*, which means 'to use, make use of, avail one's self of, employ, apply, enjoy, etc." When the government takes

property and gives it to a private individual, and the public has no right to use the property, it strains language to say that the public is "employing" [using] the property, regardless of the incidental benefits that might accrue to the public from the private use. The term "public use," then, means that either the government or its citizens as a whole must actually "employ" [use] the taken property....

Tellingly, the phrase "public use" contrasts with the very different phrase "general Welfare" used elsewhere in the Constitution.... The Constitution's text, in short, suggests that the Takings Clause authorizes the taking of property only if the public has a right to employ [use] it, not if the public realizes any conceivable benefit from the taking....

The consequences of today's decision are not difficult to predict, and promise to be harmful.... Allowing the government to take property solely for public purposes is bad enough, but extending the concept of public purpose to encompass any economically beneficial goal guarantees that these losses will fall disproportionately on poor communities.[6]

Justice Thomas warns this burden will fall most heavily on the poor—those with the fewest resources to defend themselves against government intrusion. At stake was nothing less than the private ownership of property, one of the most fundamental concepts of this republic alongside the rule of law. Even free speech is no longer free if those in power could seize a private citizen's home under the nebulously defined concept of "public benefit." Pandora's box lay open. Echoes of socialism rumbled through the streets.

How can America wake from this nightmare? Sadly, this ruling is no dream, and the present reality is more desperate than it appears. The *Kelo* decision foreshadowed how the Oregon Health Plan would impact individuals such as Barbara Wagner. Few people recognize the hidden threads that bind these events. When fully understood, *Kelo v. New London* rang as one last, great, clarion call to *We the People. This Supreme Court decision warned that liberty itself could be lost under the benign banner of "public benefit."*

Americans must recognize the commonalties shared between the Oregon Health Plan and the *Kelo* decision. In both cases the government set out to solve real problems. The state of Oregon developed the Oregon Health Plan hoping to bring healthcare to previously uninsured residents. The city of New London, Connecticut seized Susette Kelo's Victorian cottage to make room for new construction, hoping to revitalize the sluggish local economy. However, both cases perversely inverted the concept of a limited government that is "of the people, by the people, and for the people." In both cases, the welfare of government trumped the wellbeing of the individual citizen. This represents the ultimate failure of a constitutional republic.

Once the government breaches the confines of the Constitution's original intent, political power expands without limit. With time, the "greater good" of the whole replaces individual liberty. The concept of a powerful, "fixed Constitution" to which even the Supreme Court must yield is all that stands between *We the People* and tyranny.

> *Kelo v. New London rang as one last, great, clarion call to We the People. This Supreme Court decision warned that liberty itself could be lost under the benign banner of "public benefit."*

How did the voyage of the great American experiment end on these unrecognizable shores? Only by unraveling the forces that link these stunning realities can America see her future.

Finding the Tie that Binds

In the past twenty years, Americans have witnessed tremendous change in their country. Each night the evening news exposes the chaos that spans this nation. Yet, Americans absorb each devastating event as if for the first time, unaware each event is but a different face of the same process:

1) Oregon offers a woman physician-assisted suicide rather than chemotherapy.
2) The Supreme Court sweeps away property rights.
3) A prominent bioethicist advocates infanticide (the killing of infants with disabilities) to reduce the cost of healthcare.
4) The director of the Center for Medicare and Medicaid Services

states the British healthcare rationing body NICE is a "global treasure."

5) The federal government mandates that citizens purchase the services of a private industry (health insurance) simply to remain in good standing.

6) Prior to her appointment to the Supreme Court, a Judge declares the "Court of Appeals is where policy is made."

7) Following Chrysler's bankruptcy, the government violates bankruptcy law by transferring assets from secure investors to unsecure investors.[7]

8) A teacher reprimands a 13-year-old California student for drawing the American flag with the words "God Bless America" for an art class.

9) A judge finds the words "under God" in the Pledge of Allegiance unconstitutional.

10) North Carolina considered altering its 11th grade curriculum to not teach American history before 1877, thus eliminating the Founding Fathers worldview.[8]

America stands at a pivotal moment; the decisions made over the next several years will greatly determine which of two possible futures will become reality. To one side stands the heritage of *American freedom*, hewn from the wilderness and sculpted by the worldview of our Founding Fathers. This political philosophy argues that a limited government under the constraint of the "Fixed Truth" of the Constitution's original intent best secures individual liberty. This worldview undergirds the thinking of traditional conservative thought, perhaps seen most visibly in today's 9.12 Projects and the massive Tea Party movement.

In opposition stands the worldview of postmodern thought where individual autonomy is the basis for truth: truth is what is true for you; truth is what is true for me. For these individuals complete autonomy *is* freedom; in fact, *autonomous freedom* defines what it means to be American. For the postmodern thinker, *restraint* of behavior *is* the evil of our day. What could bring more freedom than a world without boundaries? What is more nonconfrontational than a world where no one idea carries more weight than another? What is more peaceful than a world without moral judgment? This worldview undergirds the thinking of today's secular progressive movement.

On the surface, these two political philosophies appear similar in that both strive for "freedom." However, their similarity is short lived; at their roots they are polar opposites. The former holds to the concept of the "Fixed Truths" of the "laws of nature and of nature's God" as found in the *Declaration of Independence*. The latter maintains that claiming to know the "Truth" represents the height of arrogance. The first believes in the possibility of American exceptionalism, that America can indeed be the shining city on a hill that President Reagan so passionately spoke of; the second believes that to say America should lead world events in the pursuit of liberty is little more than vain conceit. One believes it is possible to fight a just and noble war. The other believes war is an imposition of will; this fact alone makes war evil in every circumstance—who are we to impose our values on Iraq or Afghanistan? One stands with the great orator Edmond Burke, "Liberty too must be limited in order to be possessed."[9] The other maintains the limitation of liberty is the single greatest evil of our age.

In a confusing blur of political spin, our Founding Fathers' concept of "fixed Truth" is demonized as dangerous extremism while the worldview of relative truth is lauded as the pinnacle of human progress. Americans are left uncertain about what to believe. Amidst this confusion, postmodern thought quietly masquerades as the great liberator.

What happens to the foundations of freedom when postmodern thought destroys the concept of a "Fixed Truth"? As existentialist thinker Jean-Paul Sartre (1905-1980) once noted, *no finite point has meaning unless it has an infinite point of reference.*[10] Without a fixed point of reference even the concept of freedom loses meaning.

History teaches us that freedom without form breeds chaos, and when chaos has destroyed order, the yearning for order will destroy true freedom.[11] When the basis of true liberty is destroyed, a new kind of freedom emerges that

> But what happens to the foundations of freedom when postmodern thought destroys the concept of a "Fixed Truth"? When the basis of true liberty is destroyed, a new kind of freedom emerges that knows no bounds. Private property is no longer protected by the Constitution. Individual liberty subjugated to the "greater good" of society.

knows no bounds. *We the People* find the private ownership of property no longer protected by the Constitution. *We the People* find individual liberty subjugated to the "greater good" of society, even if this means replacing chemotherapy with physician-assisted suicide.

America's struggle to find a dominant worldview drives today's explosive culture war. This struggle surfaces on multiple fronts: healthcare, Supreme Court appointments, education, and foreign policy. *The Battle for America's Soul* traces the long and passionate history of both worldviews and applies them to each of these current issues. Only when Americans fully understand the deep and powerful forces driving these two fundamentally opposing philosophies will they understand the full fury of today's culture war. Only when Americans know their history can they envision their future.

There is flow to history. A progression of thought is sweeping this nation into an age where Americans are witnessing the death of Truth. When Truth dies, the repercussions on Reason itself will be nothing short of titanic. When Truth dies, Reason will become non-reason and America will be forever changed. *For as we think, so we are.*

Whoever controls the concept of truth controls power. By changing the concept of Truth, postmodern thought erodes the philosophical foundations of freedom. Americans can see this most clearly in *Kelo v. New London.* Using postmodern thought five Supreme Court Justices determined what the Constitution meant for them. Using traditional thought four Justices dissented bitterly asserting the Constitution's meaning was fixed. By a single vote, the new truth of "public benefit" (the personal view of five Justices) replaced the fixed truth of "public use" (the actual words of the Fifth Amendment of the U.S. Constitution).

When Supreme Court Justices gain power to alter the original intent of the Constitution, *We the People* cannot defend our freedoms—there is no fixed point of reference by which to measure justice. *We the People* can no longer protect our homes against seizure for private development by appealing to unwavering constitutional rights. Postmodern thought moves the bar by erasing all fixed points of reference. According to the Supreme Court, local governments can now take possession of private homes for matters of "public benefit." This marks only the beginning.

Once the standard of "public benefit" replaces the fixed points of reference that protect individual liberty, the foundations of freedom, in fact, the foundations that govern our constitutional republic, vanish. Barbara Wagner's story portrays this with stunning clarity. To quote Dr. Walter Shaffer once again, "We can't cover everything for everyone. Taxpayer dollars are limited for publicly funded programs. We try to come up with policies that provide the most good for the most people."[12] Postmodern thought inevitably ends in tyranny for one reason—it destroys the fundamental principles that protect *We the People*. Postmodern thought destroys the "Fixed Truth" of the Constitution and the rule of law. Under a postmodern worldview, society replaces individuality.

The Battle for America's Soul looks at America's culture war through the prism of history. It provides a lens through which America can see what is yet to come. While many images remain unclear, some come into focus. Infanticide, the active killing of infants up to four weeks of age, is one such ghost rising from the ashes of ancient Greece. Unthinkable? Prior to June 23, 2005, the fact that local governments could seize private property with the blessing of the Supreme Court was unthinkable. Today it stands as settled case law. Before June of 2008 the fact that a state government would refuse a patient chemotherapy and offer physician-assisted suicide in its place was unfathomable. Yet Barbara Wagner could swear to its reality, had she lived to tell her story.

The following chapter will show why America's current path will inevitably lead to a culture that condones the killing of infants with disabilities. As unrelated as infanticide and property rights may appear, they are inextricably linked by a common underlying *worldview*—this is the tie that binds.

Notes

1   Barbara Wagner, KVAL, Report by Susan Harding, July 31, 2008, http://www.kval.com/news/26140519.html
2   Walter Shaffer, World Net Daily, June 19, 2008, http://www.worldnetdaily.com/index.php?fa=PAGE.view&pageId=67565
3   Som Saha, KVAL, Report by Susan Harding, July 31, 2008
4   Barbara Wagner, World Net Daily, June 19, 2008
5   Gerald Ford, Presidential Address to a joint session of Congress, 12 August, 1974.

6   Clarence Thomas, Kelo v. New London/Dissent, June 23, 2005, http://en.wikisource.org/wiki/Kelo_v._New_London/Dissent_Thomas

7   Michael Barone, "White House Puts UAW Ahead of Property Rights," The Examiner, May 6, 2009. http://www.washingtonexaminer.com/politics/White-House-puts-UAW-ahead-of-property-rights-44415057.html

8   Molly Henneberg, "North Carolina Schools May Cut Chunk Out of U.S. History Lessons," FOXNews.com, February 3, 2010. http://www.foxnews.com/us/2010/02/03/north-carolina-schools-cut-chunk-history-lessons/

9   Edmond Burke, *Letter to the Sheriffs of Bristol*, (1777), *The Oxford Dictionary of Quotations,* (Oxford & New York: Oxford University Press, Revised Fourth Edition, 1996), p. 157.

10 Francis Schaeffer, *The Complete Works of Francis Schaeffer Volume 1: He is There and Not Silent*, (Westchester, Illinois: Crossway Books, 1988), pp. 277-278.

11 Eric Hoffer wrote, "When freedom destroys order, the yearning for order will destroy freedom."

12 Walter Shaffer, World Net Daily, June 19, 2008, http://www.worldnetdaily.com/index.php?fa=PAGE.view&pageId=67565

CHAPTER TWO

WE THE PEOPLE V. THE STATE

History is a gallery of pictures
in which there are few originals and many copies.
Alexis de Tocqueville (1805-1859)

The unforgiving stainless steel counter top of the soiled utility room pressed against his back. John struggled to breathe, lungs burning as weak muscles pulled hard against the air. His obliquely set eyes searched the room. Why did the doctor not give him oxygen? His heart pounded. Where was the pediatrician with the ventilator? Why did everyone leave? Pinned under the carelessly bound sheet, John's little arms tensed rhythmically as he gasped for air. Cold crept into his tiny, premature body.

Moved by John's feeble cry, Jill swathed him in a small, soft blanket. For 45 minutes he basked under her tender touch. With knowing gaze, Jill examined John's short neck and flattened nasal bridge; they betrayed an extra 21st chromosome. Indeed, John had Down's syndrome. With the calm of a nurse who knew death drew near, Jill rocked him gently. Her breath warmed his cheek. Periodically she held him against the light, peering through paper-thin skin to see if John's tiny heart was still beating. Soon the work of breathing proved too much for John's underdeveloped lungs. His heart slowed, then stopped. John Doe's short life ended. His struggle was over.

The physician never intended for John to live. Infants rarely survive late-term, induced-labor abortions. Like other John Does before him, the failed procedure left John in a world meant for neither the living nor the dead. Accidentally born alive, these infants are left to die from asphyxiation, oftentimes on a stainless steel counter top of a soiled utility room. The ancients of classical Greece called this "exposure"—killing infants by exposing them to conditions they were certain not to survive. Jill knew of another John Doe at Christ Hospital in Oak Lawn, Illinois who fought to live for nearly eight hours before drawing his last breath.

This story briefly emerged in the national press during the 2008 Presidential campaign. In response to the infanticide at Christ Hospital, the Illinois Born-Alive Infants Protection Act sought to mandate medical care for infants such as John. While in the Illinois State Senate, Barack Obama opposed this legislation. This story raises at least three questions:

1) Should all newborn infants receive medical care? Even if born with a disability?
2) What does Barack Obama's opposition to the Illinois Born-Alive Infants Protection Act reveal about his worldview?
3) Is this an isolated story or does the death of John Doe reflect the larger battle between the wellbeing of the individual and the greater good of society?

Infanticide Reborn at Princeton University

When asked to contemplate the killing of newborn children, most people think of a far-off land somewhere in the distant past. Images of ancient Greece come to mind. That some might advocate for such a practice in America is utterly unthinkable. However, infanticide was reborn when Princeton University's Chair of bioethics, Peter Singer, launched himself into the international spotlight by boldly championing the usefulness of this ancient practice. What did he say that brought such notoriety? Excerpts from two of his books speak for themselves:

> We think that some infants with severe disabilities should be killed... This recommendation may cause particular offense to readers who were themselves born with disabilities,

perhaps even the same disabilities we are discussing… For reasons given later in this book, decisions whether infants should live or die are very different from life and death decisions in the case of people who can understand, or once were capable of understanding, at least some aspects of what a decision to live or die might mean.[1,2]

There remains, however, the problem of the lack of any clear boundary between the newborn infant, who is clearly not a person in the ethically relevant sense, and the young child, who is. In our book, *Should the Baby Live?*, my colleague Helga Kuhse and I suggested that a period of twenty-eight days after birth might be allowed before the infant is accepted as having the same right to life as others. This is clearly before the infant could have a sense of its own existence over time, and would allow a couple to decide that it is better not to continue with a life that has begun very badly.[3]

Infanticide in America? Can this really be the Chair of Bioethics at Princeton speaking? With these statements Peter Singer turned the clock back nearly two millennia. The rise of Hippocratic medicine in late antiquity banished infanticide. However, with the dawning of the 21st century, the killing of unwanted infants (up to 28 days after they are born) threatens to write itself into the pages of American medicine. In an age of limited resources and unlimited demand, the infanticide of children born with disabilities offers the prospect of cost effective medicine. Avoiding the expensive care needed for infants with disabilities frees healthcare dollars for the treatment of children more gifted. While shocking, Singer's point rings true: this is "cost effective healthcare."

In the story of Barbara Wagner, Americans witnessed the first offer of government-sponsored euthanasia within the United States. Now, from inside the ivory towers of academia and the polished corridors of Christ Hospital, infanticide knocks on the door of cultural acceptability. This begs the question, "What do these stories have to do with the future of American healthcare?" The answer? Everything.

With time, the unthinkable becomes thinkable; with more time, the thinkable becomes accepted. This is the nature of culture. This is the experience of western civilization. Without a fixed point of reference, social mores drift down the river of the ages. As time presses forward, each idea folds into the next, *creating flow to history.* By tracing this flow through the centuries, details sharpen in the light of new perspective. When linked by commonalities in thought, patterns emerge from the shadows of the past. Ideas recycle with remarkable consistency, at times nearly verbatim.

Because each worldview—each understanding of the concept of Truth— inevitably leads to its own logical conclusions regardless of the century, many of the debates in culture today also appear in the archives of history. This holds true for both euthanasia and infanticide.

America is not the first to struggle with the role of the physician in society. History reveals what happens when cultures place physicians under the powerful hand of government. Alexis de Tocqueville noted, *"History is a gallery of pictures in which there are few originals and many copies."*[4] Only by knowing the past can one see the future.

The Future of American Healthcare

As I neared completion of my internal medicine training in the late 1990's, I wanted to look into the future of American healthcare. Shocked by the statements of one of the most prominent American bioethicists of our time, I set out to understand how modern culture could consider reviving the archaic procedure of infanticide. At the time I began my research, that Oregon would soon offer a citizen State-sponsored euthanasia remained unthinkable.

My studies included numerous courses on classical philosophy, ancient Greek and Roman culture, the annals of great ideas, the history of freedom, and the foundations of American constitutionalism. I read some sixty thousand of pages of source material spanning the disciplines of history, philosophy, science, ethics, and law. Beginning with Plato and Hippocrates, I worked my way through the ages, seeking the hidden links that bind the story of human thought. As I studied the evidence, fascinating patterns emerged.

For the past 2,500 years physicians have served only one of two possible roles in western culture. They either follow Hippocrates, devoting themselves to serve the individual patient or they follow Plato, functioning as servants of the State. Though poorly understood, these two archetypal views form the true foundation of today's healthcare debate.

My research not only provided insight into the future of American healthcare, it unraveled the mystery of America's cultural divide. *The Battle for America's Soul* unmasks the reshaping of America and reveals the threads that bind seemingly dissimilar events together. Issues such as the radical nature of the Oregon Health Plan, the stunning decision of *Kelo v. New London*, the infanticide of John Doe, the government's violation of bankruptcy law in dealing with Chrysler, and the failure of America's public schools all reflect different faces of a single process.

Two dominant worldviews struggle for control of America. One empowers and protects the individual; one surrenders power to the State. We the People must understand this battle of worldviews if individual liberty is to survive. We the People must understand this battle of worldviews if individual liberty is to survive.

This book walks the reader through history, portraying its lessons, not as separate stories but as ongoing skirmishes in an epic battle of worldviews. It allows Americans who love this great nation to understand the apparent insanity that surrounds them. By understanding *how* people think, *what* they think becomes disturbingly clear.

Two dominant worldviews struggle for control of America. One empowers and protects the individual; one surrenders power to the State. We the People must understand this battle of worldviews if individual liberty is to survive. Walk with me down this road less traveled.

Your Heart is not Your Own

In January of 2008 British Prime Minister Gordon Brown supported legislation giving hospitals the right—without prior consent from the patient or their family—to automatically harvest organs from patients who died. Under this legislation, hospitals assume patients wish to be organ donors unless either they previously removed their name from the national registry or a family member expressly objected. To encourage this practice, the government planned to "rate" hospitals on how many patients they "converted" into organ donors.[5] This form of "governmental oversight" under a national health service pressures physicians to secure organs for their hospitals, even without the knowledge of either patients or families.

As in America, Britain lacks enough organs to treat the many patients needing new hearts, lungs, livers, or kidneys. Approximately 1,000 Brits die each year awaiting transplant surgery. Increasing the number of organs available for transplantation by harvesting them without explicit consent would shorten the waiting list. As a result, Prime Minister Brown endorsed this proposal to save lives. In this sense, one might even consider his effort to pass this legislation noble.

However, a number of questions arise. After someone dies, whose interests are of primary concern? The deceased patient? The family? Or should the State harvest organs needed for the "greater good" of society even without the family's consent? Does the "public benefit" of this program make it acceptable? In the Supreme Court ruling of *Kelo v. New London* the words "public benefit" spelled the loss of liberty for Susette Kelo.

When examined closely, no matter how well intended the motives, each of these cases lies under the cold shadow of socialism. In each case, the State stepped in to "do good" for the majority of its citizens. But in the end, the State sacrificed individual liberty on the altar of the "social good" with chilling consistency.

> In each case, the State stepped in to "do good" for the majority of its citizens. But in each case, the State sacrificed individual liberty on the altar of the "social good" with chilling consistency.

For Barbara Wagner, the state of Oregon denied her treatment, instead allocating resources for other citizens who could be treated "more effectively." For Susette Kelo, the city of New London seized her home to generate economic growth for the community. For Peter Singer, society should sacrifice infants with disabilities in order to free up funds for the routine health care of more gifted children. For Prime Minister Brown, legislation that aggressively promoted the harvesting of organs from deceased patients, even without their consent, would help the 8,000 people waiting on the transplant list.

History has seen this before. "From each according to his ability, to each according to his need." Karl Marx believed every person should contribute to society whatever he or she was able; in return, the State provided basic care for its citizens. However, when Marx said "From each according to his ability" did he mean a person's life? Home? Heart? Child if he or she was born with a disability? As a nation whose forefathers gave their lives for the love of individual liberty and fought for the privilege of personal freedom, how did America come to this?

America stands at a threshold of deep-seated change in culture. Washington passed massive healthcare legislation against the will of the American people. Six months after President Obama signed healthcare reform legislation into law, 61% of likely voters wanted the law repealed, including 50% who strongly favored repeal. Only 33% of likely voters wanted the law left in place.[6] The unprecedented force and political gamesmanship used to pass "healthcare reform" shocked the American people.

However, *We the People* elected these men and women to office. In doing so, *We the People* laid our liberties at the doorstep of government. French writer Josephe de Maistre once noted, "Every country has the government it deserves."[7] One central question faces America today: What kind of government will this be?

Healthcare reform in light of history: We have been here before

The Legacy of Hippocrates

The year—1871. Surrounded by western Turkey's windswept plains, archeologist Heinrich Schliemann watched his childhood dream unfold. Using the writings of Homer, Schliemann finally discovered what he believed to be the lost city of Troy just inland from the turquoise waters of the Aegean Sea. Continuing the dig, archeologists unearthed nine cities, each built upon the rubble of the one before. This new evidence suggested that Troy lay desolate for nearly 400 years after the seventh city was burned in 1180 B.C., possibly the result of Homer's Trojan War.

Portions of ancient Greek literature are a fascinating blend of history and mythology. For example, Homer wrote about a Greek physician named Asclepius whose two sons fought with the Spartans at Troy. The Trojans killed his first son, Machaon, when the Spartans smuggled him into the ancient city with an elite band of warriors aboard the famed Trojan Horse. The second son, Podalirius, lost his way when returning home after the war. Podalirius eventually settled on the southwestern coast of Asia Minor in the city of Syrne where he practiced medicine, the profession of his father.

In ancient Greece, the art of medicine survived by passing skills from father to son. When the descendents of Podalirius split several generations later, one branch settled on the Greek island of Cos. There a visionary arose destined to alter the face of Western medicine forever.

Born in 460 B.C., Hippocrates of Cos rapidly rose to assume the honor of the most famous member of the Asclepiads, the family of physicians revered since the Trojan War. Both Plato and Aristotle wrote of Hippocrates with great respect. This Father of Medicine's contributions have lasted nearly two and a half millennia. Hippocrates steered the focus of the physician toward the afflicted patient. He also paved the way for the scientific method in medicine emphasizing observation, attention to detail, and treatment based on these findings.

Hippocrates' greatest contribution to western civilization set a patient-centered standard for medical ethics. Though some historians argue that Hippocrates did not write much of the Hippocratic Corpus himself, none debate its profound impact.[8] Hippocratic medicine emphasized several concepts, however, the "greater good" of society held no place in Hippocratic thought. The physician's commitment to the well-being of the individual patient formed the central theme of Hippocratic medicine:

1) "*Primum non nocere*—First, do no harm."[9] This powerful statement served as the bedrock of Hippocrates' medical ethic. Though written nearly 2,500 years ago, "First do no harm" concisely articulates the American expectation of modern medicine.

2) "The physician sees terrible things, touches what is loathsome, and from others' misfortunes harvests troubles of his own."[10] Quoting Hippocrates, twentieth century historian Oswei Temkin recalled the lifelong commitment of a physician to the patients' highest good even at considerable personal expense.

3) "For if love of men is present, love of the art is also present."[11] Quoting Hippocrates, Temkin wrote of the Hippocratic physician's love for the patient.

4) "I will not give poison to anyone though asked to do so, nor will I

suggest such a plan. Similarly I will not give a pessary to a woman to cause abortion. But in purity and in holiness I will guard my life and my art."[12] The Hippocratic Oath itself memorialized the sanctity of life from conception to natural death.

Ancient medicine struggled with the lack of adequate treatment for severe pain. Some patients who preferred voluntary death to ongoing agony requested that physicians provide medications to commit suicide. In this context "I will not give poison to anyone though asked to do so" gives insight into Hippocrates' underlying philosophy. Even when faced with a patient's uncontrolled pain, Hippocrates refused to participate in physician-assisted suicide.

5) "In name there are many doctors, but in fact there are very few."[13] Again quoting Hippocrates, Temkin noted the rarity of the truly excellent physician.

6) Ludwig Edelstein quoted the ancient Greek physician and anatomical scholar, Erasistratus, to demonstrate the high moral calling of the physician:

> Most fortunate indeed, wherever it happens that the physician is both, perfect in his art and most excellent in his moral conduct. But if one of the two should have to be missing, then it is better to be a good man devoid of learning than to be a perfect practitioner of bad moral conduct, and an untrustworthy man—if indeed it is true that good morals compensate for what is missing in art, while bad morals can corrupt and confound even perfect art.[14]

7). Temkin described how Hippocrates distanced the practice of medicine from monetary reimbursement:

> He values his reputation, and he claims a right to his fee. But whenever the need arises, his concern for the fee must yield to consideration for the patient's welfare. He does not worry his sick patients by arguing about his fee; he considers their circumstances and their means, and even assists aliens

who lack resources. Nor is he so hardened as to refuse help to recalcitrant patients.[15]

Not only did these new standards set the Hippocratic physician apart in the ancient world, they framed the bedrock of modern medicine in America. Where did they come from? To frame this moral code, Hippocrates turned to his worldview, that of a Pythagorean philosopher.

The Lasting Influence of Pythagoras

The writings of Ludwig Edelstein open a wealth of understanding to the worldview of Hippocrates. Edelstein, a twentieth century master scholar and historian, devoted his life to the study of ancient medicine, philosophy, and classical philology. In particular he loved the giants of ancient Greece.

Edelstein believed that physicians received their scientific instruction from the philosophers—rather than the philosopher from the physician—grounding medical science on a strong philosophical (rather than a purely scientific) base. He argued that Hippocrates followed Pythagorean philosophy, devoting himself to the school of thought founded by the early Greek mathematician and philosopher Pythagoras (582-496 B.C.).[16]

Hippocrates and his Pythagorean counterparts found themselves in the minority of Greek thought with respect to their views on human life.[17] Their principles separated them from the cultural and philosophical norms of the day.[18] In ancient Greece, the practices of physician-assisted suicide, abortion, infanticide, and euthanasia were common,[19] and at times, even socially encouraged. Edelstein wrote:

> Ancient religion did not proscribe suicide. It did not know of any eternal punishment for those who voluntarily ended their lives. Likewise it remained indifferent to feoticide [abortion]. Its tenets did not include… an immortal soul for which men must render account to their Creator. Law and religion left the physician free to do whatever seemed the best to him.[20]

Most of the Greek philosophers even commended abortion. For Plato, feoticide [abortion] is one of the regular institutions of the ideal state. Whenever the parents are beyond that age which he thinks best for the begetting of children, the embryo should be destroyed. Aristotle reckons abortion the best procedure to keep the population within the limits which he considers essential for a well-ordered community. [21]

Hippocrates and the Pythagoreans challenged this culture, creating a tradition that defined Western medicine through the late 20th century. At the center of this challenge lay the conviction that human life held intrinsic value. Pythagoreans considered human life sacred, with meaning derived from a divine source. This belief influenced their views on suicide, abortion, infanticide, and euthanasia leading them to oppose the cultural norms of the day. Edelstein explained:

It was different for Pythagoreans. They held that the embryo was an animate being from the moment of conception. That they did so is expressly attested by a writer of the third century A.D. [Galen is footnoted in Greek]... Consequently, for the Pythagoreans, abortion, whenever practiced, meant destruction of a living being. [22]

For indeed among all Greek thinkers the Pythagoreans alone outlawed suicide and did so without qualification... Moreover, for the Pythagorean, suicide was a sin against god who had allocated to man his position in life as a post to be held and to be defended. [23]

These ideas distinguished Pythagorean philosophers from their surrounding culture; these basic tenets also framed the worldview from which Hippocrates derived his Oath. Hippocrates believed the Divine gave meaning and value to human life ("suicide was a sin against the gods who had allocated to man his position in life as a post to be held and to be defended"). This divinely inspired intrinsic value of the individual patient lay at the center of Hippocratic medicine.

Recall Supreme Court Justice Clarence Thomas believed law must submit to the Fixed Truth of the Constitution. In a similar fashion, Hippocrates believed the physician must submit to the Fixed Truth of divine law (for Hippocrates, this came from the ancient gods of Greece). Under a worldview that acknowledged a higher law, neither the physician nor the State held the power to lift a hand against the patient or the citizen.

The World of Plato

Hippocrates challenged his culture creating a tradition that defined Western medicine through the late 20th century. The conviction that human life held intrinsic value was central to his thinking.

Clearly a genius of his time, Plato's (429-347 B.C.) writings shaped western civilization for centuries to follow. As student of Socrates and mentor to Aristotle, he walked with the philosophical giants of world history. Even though he was born thirty-one years after Hippocrates, Plato's views on the value of human life reflected the culture of fifth century B.C. Greece. Centuries passed before western culture felt the full impact of Hippocratic ideals.

The most famous and influential of Plato's works is his *Republic*. Translator Robin Waterfield shed light on the significance of the title in his introduction:

> The title *Republic* is a bad translation of the Greek *politeia*... *Politeia* is the public and political life of a community; in Latin this is *res publica*, 'public business'; Greek works used to be referred to by their Latin or Latinized titles: hence *Republic*. The book, however, is not by any stretch of the imagination a treatise on republicanism or Republicanism. Nevertheless, the title is immovable.
>
> In this translation, Republic is about morality—what it is and how it fulfils one's life as a human being.[24]

In Plato's world the city-state (*polis*) concerned the average citizen far more than national Greece. Athens and Sparta, the two most prominent city-states, controlled the lands around them. Athens and Sparta repeatedly formed and broke alliances with each other in an ever shifting balance of power. At times they sought regional dominance; at times they sought mutual safety. Waterfield notes that Athenian-style democracies expected every male citizen to participate in the decision making process of his community. Local citizens made decisions about the community's welfare, not elected officials who lived hundreds of miles away. Plato's *Republic* makes more sense in this context as it reflects the life of the community.

A sprawling work, the *Republic* takes the form of a dialog between Plato (using the voice of Socrates) and various friends. Plato discussed numerous subjects, concentrating on the function of the community and the fulfillment of its people. He outlined his views on the ideal *polis*. In Plato's utopia, political power did not rest with the people—power lay with the ruling elite, a governing body of philosopher kings. Plato considered philosophers the most qualified people to govern; the common citizen dutifully lived under their rule. While the elite defined the value of life, Plato believed the meaning of life came from the gods.

In his *Republic*, Plato attempted to show that morality (often translated as justice) benefited the individual as well as the broader community. The pursuit of morality provided the source of true personal happiness in what Waterfield called Plato's "assimilation into god."

Plato's *Republic* provides a somewhat lengthy and rather remarkable discussion of "god." Surprisingly, in the midst of rampant Greek polytheism, Plato spoke of god in a monotheistic sense. He believed god to be single, uniform, good, unchanging, and eternal.[25] Plato's concept of a single, supreme, yet unknown god may have inspired Paul of Tarsus when he spoke to the men at Athens 400 years later. "Men of Athens! I see that in every way you are very religious. For as I walked around and looked carefully at your objects of worship, I even found an altar with this inscription: 'To An Unknown God'."[26]

Plato believed the youth of Athens must love virtue.[27] Indeed, the *Republic* sought justice. However, Plato struggled to find the *source* of virtue and justice; the known Greek gods were not big enough. *The Greek gods were more glorified humanity than personal deity.* Asclepius, the Greek god of Medicine, provides a perfect example.

The descendants of the physician Asclepius (the man noted above whose sons fought in the Trojan War) included Podalirius and the famed Hippocrates of Cos, real historical men. However, Asclepius the Greek god of medicine, was the son of Apollo, the grandson of Zeus, and trained by the mythical Centaur Chiron. This blending of history and mythology left Plato lacking what the American Founding Fathers called the "laws of nature and of nature's God." Because Plato worked without a "higher law," he followed whatever self-evident understanding of virtue, justice, and morality he could generate independently. The only god big enough to supply the "laws of nature and of nature's God" remained unknown. The gods he knew left no *fixed moral code*. The good of the state (the greater good of society) became Plato's underlying assumption.

Absent a higher law to which he was subject Plato's philosopher king determined the value of human life. This opened the door for euthanasia to be an integral part of his polis.

However different their philosophies, Plato wrote warmly of the Pythagoreans.[28] In 388 B.C. Plato visited Archytas, his friend and powerful political figure. Even though Archytas followed Pythagorean philosophy, their opposing ideas remained in the gentlemen's court of intellectual debate.[29] Plato never specifically wrote in response to Hippocrates or the medical ethics of the Pythagoreans. However, in *Republic* he did discuss the infirm and the role of the ideal physician in some detail:

> ...but bodies which disease had penetrated through and through [the physician] would not have attempted to cure... he did not want to lengthen out good-for-nothing lives, or to have weak fathers begetting weaker sons;—if a man was not able to live in the ordinary way [the physician] had no business to cure him; for such a cure would have been of no use either to himself, or to the State.[30]

Three pages later he clarified this in a dialog with a friend:

36

"So at the same time as legislating for this type of legal practice in our community, you'll also legislate for the kind of medical practice we described. These two practices will treat the bodies and minds of those of your citizens who are naturally well endowed in these respects; as for the rest, those with a poor physical constitution will be allowed to die, and those with irredeemably rotten minds will be put to death. Right?"

"Yes, we've shown that this is the best course," he said, "for those at the receiving end of the treatment as well as for the community.[31]

The similarities between these statements and the statements of Princeton's bioethicist, Peter Singer, are beyond striking. Both believed society should sacrifice some individuals for the good of the whole. Singer addressed infants with deformities while Plato spoke to adults with disease, but their logic remains identical. One might think these men were office colleagues, not separated by more than two thousand years.

Why the resemblance? Again, the link lies in the similarity of their worldviews.

The Foundations of Two Worldviews

This discussion of ancient history lays the foundations and the importance of two diametrically opposed worldviews. On one side stand the Pythagoreans and Hippocratic physicians, where the intrinsic worth of the individual was rooted in deity and not subject to human opinion. Because of this philosophical base, neither the physician nor the government possessed the power to strip patients of their intrinsic value. These convictions set ethical standards for medicine. As noted in the Hippocratic Oath, "but in purity and in holiness I will guard my life and my art." A higher moral law that recognized the intrinsic worth of every human life held physicians and government in check. This worldview framed an ethical code for medicine that lasted nearly 2,500 years.

The worldview of Hippocrates foreshadowed the American *Declaration of Independence* in 1776:

> We hold these truths to be self-evident, that all men are created equal, that they are endowed by their Creator with certain unalienable Rights, that among these are Life, Liberty and the pursuit of Happiness.[32]

Both Hippocrates and the *Declaration of Independence* appealed to a deity to ground the basic rights of man. Similar to Supreme Court Justice Clarence Thomas in the *Kelo v. New London* decision, Hippocrates believed in a "Fixed Truth." Neither man nor government could strip an individual of his or her rights. Justice Thomas appealed to the "Fixed Truth" of the Constitution; Hippocrates appealed to the "Fixed Truth" of the Pythagorean gods. The concept of a fixed point of reference insured that medicine would always serve the patient, and government would always serve the citizen.

On the other side lay mainstream ancient culture and the dominant Greek philosophy. Decision-making with respect to the value of human life was not accountable to the gods. Absent a higher law to which he was subject, Plato's philosopher king determined the value of human life. The fact Plato pursued God and a moral life proved insufficient. The mere *desire* for a moral life did not provide a moral law to which Plato must submit. Plato possessed *no fixed points of reference*. As a result, he had no basis for the intrinsic value of human dignity. This opened the door for infanticide and euthanasia to be an integral part of his *polis* when these served to advance the "greater good," *i.e.* the welfare of the State.

The way Plato's worldview shaped his thinking on medical ethics foreshadowed the French *Declaration of the Rights of Man* in 1789:

> The representatives of the French people, organized as a National Assembly, believing that the ignorance, neglect, or contempt of the rights of man are the sole cause of public calamities and of the corruption of governments, have determined to set forth in a solemn declaration.... Therefore

the National Assembly recognizes and proclaims... the following rights of man and of the citizen:[33]

Both Plato and the French *Declaration of the Rights of Man* appeal to those in power—the philosopher king and the National Assembly respectively—for the basic rights of its citizens. However, both Plato and the French left those in power to define law as they saw fit because neither accepted the concept of a higher moral code fixed by the existence of the divine. Hence, a change in power opened the door for a change of one's basic rights. In other words, under this worldview individual rights were no longer unalienable. They were dependent on the goodwill of government.

With the *Kelo* decision, American citizens witnessed a version of this dependence on the ruling elite in the United States. Informed by a worldview nearly identical to Plato, five Supreme Court Justices used postmodern thought to violate the Constitution's original intent—and Susette Kelo lost her home.

> *The concept of a fixed point of reference insured that medicine would always serve the patient, and government would always serve the citizen. Neither the physician nor the government could strip individuals of their unalienable rights.*

The stories of Barbara Wagner, Susette Kelo, Peter Singer, Prime Minister Brown, Hippocrates, and Plato present a central struggle of the ages—the eternal tension between the good of the individual vs. the welfare of the State. Repeatedly individuals lose liberty when those in power are free to determine "truth and justice" for society, leaving individual citizens dependant on the generosity of government. Repeatedly individuals retain liberty when the individual can appeal to a fixed Truth, to an authority greater than those who hold power.

This is the fundamental Law of Liberty: Whoever controls the concept of Truth controls power. This law fuels the intense emotion behind America's culture war. A government restrained by a higher law (the laws of nature and of nature's God) allows for individual freedom; a government free to impose its will on the people—even under the banner of public benefit—ends in tyranny. *If America loses her concept of a fixed point of reference, she will assuredly lose her most treasured possession, liberty itself.*

Notes

1   Nigel Cameron, *The New Medicine: Life and Death After Hippocrates*, (Wheaton, Illinois: Crossway Books, 1991), p. 115.

2   Helga Kuhse, Peter Singer, *Should the Baby Live?*, (Oxford & New York: Oxford University Press, 1985), p. v.

3   Peter Singer, *Rethinking Life and Death—The Collapse of Our Traditional Ethics*, (St. Martin's Griffin: New York 1994), p. 217.

4   Alexis de Tocqueville, *L' Ancien régime*, (1856, ed. J. P. Mayer, 1951) p. 89 (translated by M. W. Patterson, 1933)

5   Patrick Hennessy, Laura Donnelly, "Organs to be taken without consent," Telegraph.co.uk, April 12, 2008, http://www.telegraph.co.uk/news/1575441/Organs-to-be-taken-without-consent.html

6   Rasmussen Reports, 61% Favor Repeal of Health Care Law, September 20, 2010. http://www.rasmussenreports.com/public_content/politics/current_events/healthcare/september_2010/61_favor_repeal_of_health_care_law

7   Josephe de Maistre, *Letters et Opuscules Inédits*, Vol. 1, letter 53, August 15, 1811.

8   Ludwig Edelstein, *Ancient Medicine*, (Baltimore & London: Johns Hopkins University Press, 1987), p. 144.

9   Often thought to come from the *Oath* "First do no harm" actually is found in Hippocrates' *Epidemics*. It was originally written in Greek, but the subsequent Latin translation is most often remembered. Sherwin Nuland, *Doctors: The Biography of Medicine*, (New York: Vintage Books, 1995), pp. 15-16.

10 Owsei Temkin, *Hippocrates in a World of Pagans and Christians*, (Baltimore & London: Johns Hopkins University Press, 1991), p. 19.

11 Ibid., p. 30.

12 Nigel Cameron, *The New Medicine: Life and Death After Hippocrates*, (Wheaton, Illinois: Crossway Books, 1991), p. 25.

13 Temkin, p. 23.

14 Edelstein, p. 334.

15 Temkin, p. 32.

16 Edelstein, pp. 4-63.

17 Other authors have shown there were a few other groups with views similar to those of the Pythagoreans. Martin Arbagi, "Roe and the Hippocratic Oath," *Abortion and the Constitution: Reversing Roe v. Wade through the Courts*, edited by Horan, Grant, and Cunningham, (Washington, D.C.: Georgetown University Press, 1987), pp. 159-181.

18 Edelstein, pp. 16-19.

19 It appears that infanticide was more common than abortion primarily because of the high maternal mortality rate associated with abortions until the late

1700's. Joseph Dellapenna, "Abortion and the Law: Blackmun's Distortion of the Historical Record," *Abortion and the Constitution: Reversing Roe v. Wade through the Courts*, edited by Horan, Grant, and Cunningham, (Washington, D.C.: Georgetown University Press, 1987), pp. 145-148.

20   Edelstein, p. 16.

21   Ibid, p. 18.

22   Ibid, pp. 18-19.

23   Ibid. p. 17.

24   Robin Waterfield, *Republic*, translated by Robin Waterfield, (New York: Barnes & Noble Books, 1996), pp. xi-xii.

25   Plato, *Republic*, translated by Robin Waterfield, (New York: Barnes & Noble Books, 1996), 379a-383b, 613a-613b, pp. 73-79, 369-370.

26   Paul of Tarus, Acts 18:23, *The Holy Bible, New International Version*, (Grand Rapids, Michigan: Zondervan Bible Publishers, 1982), p. 1017.

27   William Kilpatrick, *Why Johnny Can't Tell Right from Wrong*, (New York: Simon & Schuster, 1993), p. 89.

28   Plato, *Republic*, translated by Robin Waterfield. 530d-530e, pp. 262-263.

29   Robin Waterfield, p. xiv.

30   Plato, *The Republic*, translated by Benjamin Jowett, (New York: Barnes & Noble Books, 1999), p. 93.

31   Plato, *Republic*, by Waterfield, 409e-410a, p. 111.

32   American Declaration of Independence, July 4, 1776.

33   French Delaration of the Rights of Man and of the Citizen, August 26, 1789.

CHAPTER THREE

THE WANDERING NEEDLE OF HEALTHCARE'S ETHICAL COMPASS[1]

The history of medicine is, in fact, the history of humanity itself,
with its ups and downs, its brave aspirations after
truth and finality, its pathetic failures.

Fielding Garrison (1870-1935)

On November 4, 2008 America moved one step closer toward the world of Plato. Washington became the second state in the nation to legalize physician-assisted suicide. By a vote of 59% to 41%, the "Evergreen State" joined its southern neighbor in the march toward the brave new postmodern world of autonomous freedom. Removing the touchstones of society grants the individual autonomous freedom. However, when culture loses its fixed points of reference, the State gains autonomy as well—and the autonomous State wields the force of law. No doubt, change is in the air.

Only three and a half years earlier, America watched the state of Florida handle a difficult case of medical ethics. In the spring of 2005 a Florida court ordered the removal of a 41-year-old woman's feeding tube against her parents' wishes. Tempers flared and rhetoric escalated as lawyers filed repeated appeals. America divided into two camps while the world awkwardly watched the last grueling weeks of Terri Schiavo's death. In the end, only doubt, grief, and questions remained; even her ashes were scattered to the wind. This public tragedy resulted in profound loss for everyone involved. There were no winners.

What were Terri's wishes? Why were her records sealed? Why was the case never given a *de novo* review despite unprecedented bipartisan involvement? Did the courts have something to cover up? As a physician who practices hospital based medicine—from critical care to inpatient hospice—I questioned why Terri was not allowed ice chips to dampen her cracked lips. Why did she not receive moist swabs to sooth her parched tongue? By concept, every hospice patient should have access to these basic comfort measures.

How should Americans process these complex and profoundly personal events? Barbara Wagner, John Doe, Terri Schiavo. The nightly news pitches story after story, moving from one to the next without context as if each just occurred for the first time. However disturbing, these complex, emotionally charged, and high profile stories hold one redeeming aspect: they push the deeper meaning of American healthcare and end of life issues squarely into public view.

Americans desperately seek to understand the sweeping healthcare legislation narrowly passed by Congress along strict party lines. Terms such as "expert advisory panels," "clinical effectiveness research," and "the Secretary shall establish" fill the 2,700 pages of legislation. After two years of intense debate, Americans still wonder what all this really means. There is no unifying framework. There is no broader context. There are no fixed points of reference from which to judge. Even one of the bill's most ardent supporters, Speaker of the House Nancy Pelosi, admitted, "We have to pass the bill so that you can find out what is in it."[2]

A year after President Obama signed the bill into law, the basic questions asked by ordinary American's remain unanswered. What is the future of American healthcare? What does it mean to be a physician? To be a patient? *We the People* must find a moral compass to answer these questions.

Defining the Poles

At times, ethical dilemmas wrench the rudder of daily medicine sending patients, families, and physicians into uncharted waters. The tragedy of Terri

Schiavo was a prime example. Americans had never dealt with a situation quite like that before. On national television, a woman with severe brain injury slowly died from dehydration without basic measures of comfort. This "real life" TV transported America to a place beyond surreal.

When faced with uncertainties in medical ethics, each person must consult a moral compass to determine where his or her needle points. To maintain orientation, Western medicine uses the concepts of *beneficence*, *nonmaleficence, autonomy*, and *justice* as "true north" for ethical navigation. Briefly defined:

1) *Beneficence* is to do good.
2) *Nonmaleficence* is to do no harm.
3) *Autonomy* is to respect patients' wishes regarding treatment options, not forcing them to undergo treatment they do not desire.
4) *Justice* is to do what is morally right.

Medical students and residents commonly learn these four concepts form the foundation of medical ethics. These touchstones guide physicians for the remainder of their careers. When faced with ethical challenges in daily practice, physicians use these concepts as a framework to make decisions.

> When faced with uncertainties in medical ethics, each person must look inward to consult his or her personal moral compass as a guide—to find where the needle of their ethical compass points.

However, on closer inspection, these concepts actually do not comprise a medical ethic; they are simply tools masquerading as such. To find the underlying medical ethic, one must return to ancient Greece and reexamine the divergent worldviews of <u>H</u>ippocrates and <u>P</u>lato. When placed side by side, the worldviews of these two men clarify many of the struggles in modern bioethics and help Americans understand the recent healthcare debate. Even more, their thinking provides an ethical compass. The question Americans must answer now is whether their needles point toward "<u>H</u>" or toward "<u>P</u>."

The writings of <u>H</u>ippocrates and <u>P</u>lato articulate opposing poles of thought. Though formulated 2,500 years ago, the writings of these two men bring surprising clarity to the most prominent dilemmas of medicine today. *By examining their positions, Americans can discover a common language for the complex discussion of medical ethics. This is essential as We the People debate national healthcare reform.*

Recall Plato transferred power to the State and used the physician as a tool to protect the interests of society. He calculated the value of a human life by determining its ability to enhance the State or improve the well being of others. Plato's ideal physician guarded the greater good of society by deciding when to let weak and infirm patients go untreated or die.

Because Plato's worldview contained no higher "laws of nature and nature's God," patients, physicians, and ultimately the State were free to determine the value of a given human life. Infanticide and euthanasia were accepted and often socially encouraged. Plato knew no higher moral code that restrained such practices. Plato placed the good of the whole over the well-being of the individual patient.

In Plato's *Republic* one finds the first example of Stateism (the greater good of the State supersedes the individual well-being of its citizens) applied to healthcare, "For such a cure would have been of no use either to himself, or to the State."[3] Plato's ideal physician treated the young, the fit, and the productive members of society, so they could return to work and make further contributions to society. Patients who burdened society—who were "of no use to the State"— were identified and dealt with accordingly.

> The worldviews of Plato and Hippocrates provide a language to let Americans discuss the complex subject of medical ethics. This is essential as We the People debate national healthcare reform.

Hippocrates rejected this view. Following in the footsteps of the Pythagoreans, Hippocrates believed human life was a gift from the gods. Infanticide and euthanasia played no part in his medical ethic. Hippocrates' theological underpinnings precluded individual judgment on the value of human life, restricting the *autonomy* of patients, physicians, and the State. For Hippocrates, the "laws of God" reigned supreme. This worldview provided a *consistent and reliable* fixed Truth under which Hippocrates' patients experienced freedom. Patients knew their well-being lay at the center of Hippocratic medicine.

Hippocrates placed the patient at the center of healthcare. The time tested phrase, "Above all else do no harm" clearly applied to the individual patient, not to the community as a whole. For Hippocrates, the "greater good" of society played no role in determining patient care.

The Struggle to Find True North

As a profession, medicine minted *beneficence, nonmaleficence, autonomy,* and *justice* as the bedrock of bioethical thought.[4] However, do these four concepts actually form a true bioethic? Do they provide clear and consistent answers to questions related to medical ethics? If they do, an individual's worldview will not alter the direction to which these concepts point. However, if these are only tools and not a true bioethic, they will inform but not provide clear direction.

1) <u>Abortion</u>: Abortion is perhaps the most emotionally and politically charged bioethical issue of the last half century. Arguments surrounding it continue to swirl as the four laws of bioethics provide little if any guidance.

The principle of *beneficence* (for the mother), *autonomy* (for the mother), and *justice* (for the State) support the pro-choice position. However, adding fetal considerations complicates the matter. Now *beneficence* (for the fetus), *autonomy* (for the fetus), and *nonmaleficence* (for the fetus) support the pro-life position. The entire debate hinges on who is considered the patient and the value assigned to the unborn human life. When balancing the mother's interests against those of the unborn, the principles of *beneficence* and *autonomy* break down completely. The interests of each party appear mutually exclusive.

Plato's worldview provided a clear and consistent answer. Plato did not accept the concept of the sanctity of life at any age. He determined human worth based upon its potential contribution to society. Plato allowed others in society to assign the value of life to a given person. The collective good was of primary importance. Under Plato's worldview abortion violated no moral code.

Hippocrates' worldview was equally clear and consistent. From a Hippocratic perspective, the intrinsic value of fetal life began at the moment of conception; all four concepts argue against abortion being part of medicine.

47

Thus the worldview, not the four laws of bioethics, determines an individual's position on abortion. This explains why abortion remains such an explosive issue. When the Supreme Court claimed jurisdiction over the abortion debate with *Roe v. Wade*, they guaranteed perpetual conflict. To rule in favor of abortion violates the worldview of those who side with Hippocrates; to rule against the right to abortion violates the worldview of those who side with Plato.

2) <u>Infanticide</u>: Once confined to the ivory towers of academia, infanticide emerged on the national stage with the writings of Peter Singer. Just a few years later America witnessed the infanticide of John Doe at Christ Hospital in Oak Lawn, Illinois in 2001.

Hippocrates' worldview remains clear and consistent on the issue of infanticide. For Hippocrates, the four concepts of *beneficence, nonmaleficence, autonomy,* and *justice,* made infanticide unthinkable. For Hippocrates, infant life was sacred. However, Singer now challenges this premise by using a strikingly Platonic approach.

In a manner reminiscent of Plato, Princeton University's chair of bioethics, Peter Singer, openly endorsed human infanticide in certain situations. He reached this conclusion by asserting that humans have no moral distinction from the rest of the animal kingdom. Singer then excluded the newborn from the protection of traditional western ethics by creating a distinction between being "human" (which the newborn infant is) and being "fully human" (which, according to Singer, the newborn infant is not). Hence, infants do not receive protected status until they reach five weeks of age. Singer then employed the concept of *justice* to support infanticide; he argued that the large sum of money spent on newborns with disabilities (who are not yet "fully human") was better spent in other areas of healthcare.

Again, the worldview, not the four "laws of bioethics," determines the conclusion. For both Plato and Peter Singer, there was no "fixed Truth" that protected an infant with disabilities. By appealing to the greater "social good" both Plato and Singer were free to kill infants who required significant amounts of healthcare. Hippocrates rejected this thinking outright.

3) <u>Euthanasia and Physician-Assisted Suicide</u>: Holding to Plato's worldview and arguing from the vantage point of *autonomy*, one may contend that a patient has the right to terminate his or her own life. This was certainly common in early Greece. Plato's understanding of *justice* (and that of the Oregon Health Plan) may even compel active State-sponsored euthanasia when the interests of the State outweigh the interests of the patient. Nazi Germany used this logic when it starved to death many of its mentally ill during a time of financial crisis.

However, physician-assisted suicide and active euthanasia lie completely outside the realm of medical practice when employing the concept of *nonmaleficence* from a Hippocratic perspective. Again the worldview—the underlying assumptions—mandates the logical conclusion.

4) <u>Equality of Treatment</u>: A study[5] released in May, 2010 revealed Texas physicians are abandoning Medicare at an alarming rate. Prior to 2007 only a handful of physicians quit taking payment from Medicare each year. In fact, between 1998 and 2002 no more than three physicians left Medicare in any given year. However, more than 300 Texas physicians have dropped Medicare in the past two years, fifty of these during the first three months of 2010. This represents a 10,000% increase in less than a decade, a most disturbing trend.

Here the concept of *justice* fails to even support itself. On one hand *justice* states that people deserve equal treatment. However, when the government provides medical care for an ever-expanding number of seniors, proponents of a *justice* argument defend lowering Medicare reimbursement given the limited government funds available. Yet, when the Washington lowers reimbursement below operating costs, physicians must limit their exposure to patients on Medicare in order to remain in practice. This results in the lack of access to healthcare for precisely the population Medicare intended to serve.

Plato's ideal physician solved this problem by assessing the individual's value to society; "...but bodies which disease had penetrated through and through [the physician] would not have attempted to cure." If

Driven by unbridled public expectation, America is rapidly approaching a time when treatment and litigation costs will exceed available resources. When this happens, the ability to maintain Hippocratic ideals becomes untenable.

the patient's contribution to society exceeded the resources required for treatment, the physician used the resources and treated the patient. If not, the physician either left the patient untreated or opted to employ physician-assisted suicide. Plato recommended limiting access to care for the weak and infirm, conditions common in an elderly population.

The trend reported in Texas reflects the single most difficult issue when confronting healthcare reform: unlimited demand in the face of limited supply. Driven by a confluence of issues, America is rapidly approaching a time when treatment, administration, and litigation costs will exceed available resources. When this happens, the ability to maintain Hippocratic ideals becomes impossible.

A 2010 Congressional Budget Office (CBO) report revealed that under President Obama's budget the total American national debt would grow from $7.5 trillion at the end of 2009 to $20.3 trillion by 2020 reaching 90% of the entire Gross Domestic Product.[6] Congressman Paul Ryan (then ranking member on the House Budget Committee) estimated that interest on this debt would skyrocket to $916 billion annually.[7] Ryan also estimated that when fully implemented, the new healthcare legislation carries a true ten-year cost of $2.6 trillion.[8] A more recent CBO report revealed our nation's deficit rose from $163 billion in 2007 to $1.3 trillion in 2010; it then projected our deficit would reach an historic high of $1.5 trillion for the 2011 fiscal year.[9]

When America can no longer pay its bills only two choices remain with respect to healthcare:

1) Follow Plato. The State will allocate healthcare according to the "cost effectiveness" of treatment. Patients who contribute to society are treated. Patients for whom care is expensive are left untreated for the sake of "greater good."

2) Follow Hippocrates. Patients and physicians can control the cost of healthcare, without government rationing, by consistently asking two questions: "How much does this cost?" and "Do we need this test or treatment?" When coupled with ending abusive medical litigation, these simple free-market questions can reduce healthcare costs, but leave healthcare

decision-making in the hands of patients and their physicians."

* * *

The concepts of *beneficence, nonmaleficence, autonomy,* and *justice* do not constitute a medical ethic in and of themselves. They are only *tools,* albeit essential tools, which require an underlying philosophy to be useful. Without a compass, these tools run aground when navigating the difficult waters of modern bioethics. Plato and Hippocrates outlined two poles of thought that have retained their relevance over the millennia. Plato took an *autonomous* view when approaching medical ethics leaving the philosopher king free to decide the "social good." Hippocrates submitted to a *higher law* leaving neither the State nor the physician free to violate the Pythagorean moral code. A review of the history of western civilization reveals no third alternative. Americans must now ask, which pole did the recent healthcare legislation move us toward? The answer becomes deeply disturbing when weighed against the scales of history.

The Wandering Needle

Although Hippocrates actually predated Plato by approximately 33 years, Plato's philosophy exemplified the social norms of the time.[10] Hippocrates challenged the status quo and so began the resulting ebb and flow that has lasted two and a half millennia.

Propelled by the adoption of Hippocratic values by early Christians, the transition from pre-Hippocratic (Platonic) thought to what we now recognize as the Hippocratic tradition took place over several hundred years.[11] For the next 2,000 years, Judeo-Christian philosophy remained a dominant force in the formation of the Western moral code, carrying Hippocratic ideals with it. By the fifth century A.D., the practice of non-Hippocratic medicine had vanished in the West.

While proponents of a Platonic worldview always existed, Western civilization largely chose the Hippocratic path. Imagine an aging patient who

---

*   'The author, Dr. C. L. Gray, founded the non-profit organization, Physicians for Reform, in 2006. Physicians for Reform uses Hippocratic principles to craft patient-centered, fiscally responsible policy. Dr. Gray seeks to address the challenges facing American healthcare, but to do so in a way that keeps the power of medical decision-making in the hands of patients and physicians, not Washington. For more information visit www.PhysiciansForReform.org

struggled with arthritis. Which physician would he or she choose to see? Plato's ideal physician who weighed the treatment options in light of what was best for the State? Or a Hippocratic physician who rendered care based on the wellbeing of the individual patient? History reveals substantial gravitation to the Hippocratic Pole. Figuratively speaking, physicians would have worn an "H" on their white coats during these many centuries. However, over the last 100 years the nearly unanimous consensus of the previous two millennia has shifted.

The ideas of Plato found new life during the late 1800's in the writings of Friedrich Nietzsche. Nietzsche set the stage for this paradigm shift in his quest for moral autonomy. He expressed his perspective of the patient/physician relationship in his book *Twilight of the Idols*:

> The invalid is a parasite on society. In a certain state it is indecent to go on living. To vegetate on in cowardly dependence on physicians and medications after the meaning of life, the *right* to life, has been lost ought to entail the profound contempt of society. Physicians, in their turn, ought to be the communicators of this contempt— not prescriptions, but every day a fresh dose of *disgust* for their patients.... To create a new responsibility, that of the physician, in all cases in which the highest interest of life, of *ascending* life, demands the most ruthless suppression and sequestration of degenerating life—for example in determining the right to reproduce, the right to be born, the right to live....[12]

This rings of Plato. Following the footprints of Nietzsche, physicians working for the Third Reich threw off all Hippocratic restraint. For example, the Dachau Hypothermia Experiments lowered subjects into ice water to see how long it would take them to freeze to death. Before they died, they were "rewarmed" using various methods. Physicians submerged some of the severely hypothermic patients in vats of hot oil or placed them under scorching lamps. For others, physicians forced scalding water into the victim's stomachs, rectums, or surgically opened abdominal cavities. All this was done to allegedly determine the optimum method for treating hypothermic pilots. (Of note, no good data were recorded from these "experiments."[13]) Sadly, scores of other examples abound. Many patients would have found a figurative "P" embroidered on the white coats of their physicians during the early 1940's.

In his book *Murderous Science*, Benno Müller-Hill recounts events in German medicine reflecting on an unholy union between physicians and the Holocaust:

> Why was it the physicians who so particularly took it upon themselves to become the theoreticians and priests of the cult of extermination? Why did doctors trained in anthropology stand on the railway ramp to Auschwitz and carry out the process of selection and killing? Why were doctors trained in psychiatry prepared to kill their patients or allow them to starve to death? It was the result of a long historical evolution. The traditional role of the priest....
>
> The white coat was their priestly garment. Physicians with anthropological and psychiatric training had acquired, on 9 March 1943, the right and duty to carry out the selection and killing of the victims. They fought hard to retain this right, and sacrificed millions on their alters, the ovens which they had erected everywhere. The corpses of the sacrificed returned the womb of the ovens. Their souls departed as smoke from the chimneys. Auschwitz was their greatest shrine.[14]

In the aftermath of this unfathomable carnage, the Hippocratic tradition again resurfaced with the founding of the World Medical Association. To prevent repetition of the medical atrocities of Hitler's regime, a committee drafted a special section of the Declaration of Geneva regarding medical ethics. It specifically intended to re-anchor western medicine to its Hippocratic mores.[15] Once again, patients found an "H" pinned to their physicians' coat.

But this comfort did not last. Under the banner of *autonomous freedom*, western culture steadily overturned its Hippocratic tradition.

Rejecting the Heritage of Hippocrates

1) The first major departure from Hippocratic precepts occurred in 1949 with the Declaration of Geneva itself. The Hippocratic Oath and the Declaration of Geneva contain obvious similarities—with one glaring difference. The Hippocratic Oath was just that, an oath, a swearing before one's God or gods to follow an unchanging set of standards for all time. *The Hippocratic Oath contained a fixed point of reference by which all else could be judged—precisely what postmodern thought destroys.* The Geneva Convention included no such oath; it merely laid out a list of standards open to revision. Revision waited with pressured impatience.

2) Before long, the World Medical Association altered the Declaration of Geneva. The document initially included the statement, "I will maintain the utmost respect for human life from the time of conception; even under threat." In the 1960's postmodern forces changed the penultimate clause read, "I will maintain the utmost respect for human life from its beginning..."[16]

3) A third reversal of Hippocratic principals came with the landmark year of 1973, the year the United States legalized abortion. Rejection of the Hippocratic ideal of the sanctity of life from conception to death marked perhaps the most profound reversal of the Oath. For the first time in 2,000 years, the physician publicly resumed Plato's dual roles of healer and arbiter of life.

With this action the Supreme Court stripped medicine of its fixed point of reference. Patients were no longer guaranteed their well-being would remain at the center of American medicine.

Curiously, Justice Blackmun extensively used Edelstein's work (as reviewed in chapter two) on the Hippocratic Oath in support of *Roe v. Wade*. Blackmun endeavored to show the sanctity of life for the unborn stemmed from a Pythagorean manifesto. By doing so, Blackmun sought to prove Hippocrates' medical ethics (including his conception of the sanctity of human life) were not intrinsic to medicine itself.[17,18] *With this action the Supreme Court stripped medicine of its fixed point of reference. Patients were no longer guaranteed their well-being would remain at the center of American medicne.*

Six years after *Roe v. Wade*, Francis Schaeffer and C. Everett Koop predicted further shifts away from Hippocratic principles when they wrote *Whatever Happened to the Human Race.* Schaeffer and Koop predicted the coming acceptance of euthanasia in American medicine. At that time the practice of infanticide remained utterly unthinkable.

4) The swing of the compass continued. In 1985 bioethicist Peter Singer moved infanticide from the unthinkable to the thinkable. In *Should the Baby Live* he wrote:

> We think that some infants with severe disabilities should be killed... This recommendation may cause particular offense to readers who were themselves born with disabilities, perhaps even the same disabilities we are discussing... For reasons given later in this book, decisions whether infants should live or die are very different from life and death decisions in the case of people who can understand, or once were capable of understanding, at least some aspects of what a decision to live or die might mean.[19,20]

With notables such as Singer reawakening thoughts of Plato and Nietzsche, the possibility that culture may accept this apparition from the past hovers at the bedside.

5) In 1994 Peter Singer moved America yet closer to the world of Plato with his book, *Rethinking Life and Death*:

> There remains, however, the problem of the lack of any clear boundary between the newborn infant, who is clearly not a person in the ethically relevant sense, and the young child, who is. In our book, *Should the Baby Live?*, my colleague Helga Kuhse and I suggested that a period of twenty-eight days after birth might be allowed before the

infant is accepted as having the same right to life as others. This is clearly before the infant could have a sense of its own existence over time, and would allow a couple to decide that it is better not to continue with a life that has begun very badly.[21]

6) In 1997 Oregon moved physician-assisted suicide from the thinkable to the accepted. With this legislation, Schaeffer and Koop's prediction became reality.[22,23]

7) In 1999 Princeton University appointed Peter Singer to the Ira W. DeCamp Chair of Bioethics, one of the most prestigious positions in the world of medical ethics. This appointment pushed Singer's thinking into the mainstream of bioethical thought.

8) In 2008 the Oregon Health Plan refused Barbara Wagner chemotherapy offering instead to pay for hospice care or physician-assisted suicide.

9) On November 4, 2008, the state of Washington legalized physician-assisted suicide moving America yet closer toward the world of Plato.

10) On January 31, 2009 *The Lancet*, a premier medical journal, published an article entitled "Principles for Allocation of Scarce Medical Interventions." In this article the Director of Bioethics at the National Institute of Health (NIH) introduced what he called the "Complete Lives System" (including figure below):[24]

> Consideration of the importance of complete lives also supports modifying the youngest-first principle by prioritizing adolescents and young adults over infants (figure). Adolescents have received substantial education and parental care, investments that will be wasted without a complete life. Infants, by contrasts, have not yet received these investments....

When implemented, the complete lives system produces a priority curve on which individuals aged between roughly 15 and 45 years get the most substantial chance [of receiving a scarce medical intervention], whereas the youngest and oldest people get chances that are attenuated (figure)....

Unlike allocation by sex or race, allocation by age is not invidious discrimination... Treating 65-year-olds because of stereotypes or falsehoods would be ageist; treating them differently because they have already had more life years is not.

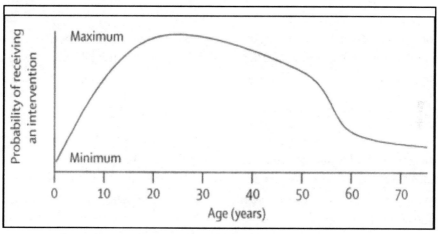

Figure: Age-based priority for receiving scarce medical interventions under the complete lives system*

With one simple graph, the Director of Bioethics at the NIH placed the thinking of Plato squarely in the highest levels of American government. Plato himself could not have expressed his thinking more concisely.

---

*   Important notes: First, as an oncologist by training, Dr. Emanuel clearly cautioned against legalizing euthanasia in the U.S. (see "Whose Right to Die," *The Atlantic*, March 1997). Second, the article and graph referenced above specifically address the allocation of scarce resources, not euthanasia. However, the concern with the Complete Lives System arises when medicine falls under government control in an age of massive deficits. In such a setting, history teaches this philosophy would spell the end of patient-centered, Hippocratic medicine here in America. The author fears that when the Patient Protection and Affordable Care Act cuts $500 billion from Medicare, nearly all healthcare resources for seniors will be considered "scarce."

Look at the graph. To the left lies the infanticide of John Doe, the little boy born with Down's Syndrome, age 0. To the right lies the offer of State-sponsored euthanasia for Barbara Wagner, age 64.

Those least able to contribute to the welfare of the State (the very young and citizens advancing in age) are the least likely to receive a medical intervention when healthcare resources are scarce. Recall America's economic forecast as determined by the non-partisan Congressional Budget Office. Recall the massive expense of the new healthcare legislation. Recall the rapid exodus of physicians from Medicare. Many medical treatments once taken for granted may soon be considered "scare."

Bioethicist Stephen Williams raised two thought provoking questions: 1) Once the heart of medicine has changed, how long will it be before compassion dries up? 2) When that happens, how long before compassion is replaced by the contempt of Nietzsche?[25] Americans must ask, did this just happen?

American Healthcare in a Postmodern World

Why the concern with history and philosophy? Because abstract worldviews find expression in everyday life, including the practice of medicine. John Doe and Barbara Wagner are not merely two unfortunate, random cases taken out of context; they represent the real world implementation of an age-old philosophy.

Once the heart of medicine has changed, how long will it be before compassion dries up? When that happens, how long before compassion is replaced by the contempt of Nietzsche?

Ideas drive behavior, even when those ideas are not given conscious expression. Even more, without understanding the concept of a worldview, events that form a clear progression of thought can masquerade as unrelated stories.

When viewed in isolation one can easily discount the stories of Barbara Wagner, Susette Kelo, Ezekiel Emanuel, and John Doe. Barbara Wagner: in any large bureaucracy one finds examples of poor communication. Susette Kelo: though unfortunate, private property remains a cornerstone of American society. Ezekiel Emanuel: the *Lancet* article represents an intellectual argument within the context of a difficult bioethical discourse. John Doe: America stands far from openly adopting infanticide.

However, when viewed though the prism of competing worldviews, these events take on new significance. They stand as warning signs to the informed citizen. Community can replace individuality; the "greater good" can replace personal liberty. Americans must understand this as they process the recently passed healthcare reform legislation. Americans, especially our senior citizens, must understand the worldview on which *The Patient Protection and Affordable Care Act* was constructed.

America must know the Director of the NIH and co-author of the "Complete Lives System" was Dr. Ezekiel Emanuel, brother of then White House Chief of Staff, Rahm Emanuel. Dr. Ezekiel Emanuel became the Special Advisor for Health Policy for President Obama and served in this role through the duration of the healthcare reform debate. One cannot escape the correlation between his "Complete Lives System" graph (see above) and the final legislation that cut $500 billion from Medicare. Given a large portion of healthcare spending occurs in the last years of life, how could one cut healthcare spending more efficiently than by limiting access to "scarce medical interventions" after the age of 60?

Without understanding the power of a worldview it is difficult to draw this conclusion. One academic paper in isolation is simply that, one academic paper in isolation. However, when weighed against the sweep of history, the thinking of Dr. Emanuel takes on new significance. His worldview aligns precisely with that of Plato, Nietzsche, and Singer. Does the fact Dr. Ezekiel Emanuel served such an influential role in crafting President Obama's signature legislation reveal anything about our President's worldview?

I once attended a lecture covering the "four laws of bioethics." Afterwards I spoke with the bioethicist giving the presentation and asked what she thought of Peter Singer's position on human infanticide. Her response was prototypically postmodern, "I don't agree with him, but I can't say that he's wrong."

Recall the definition of postmodern thought: Truth is what is true for you; Truth is what is true for me. For the postmodern thinker, *to make a moral judgment* is the evil of our day. Because the presenter shared Singer's postmodern worldview, she could say little more than, "I disagree." Sadly, this professional bioethicist was unable to state human infanticide is morally wrong; *but to condemn infanticide, one must be able to discern good from evil— the very capacity postmodern thought destroys.*

Pulled in the wake of postmodern thought even President Obama struggles with the questions of medical ethics. During the 2008 Presidential campaign, at the time of the Saddleback Church forum in Lake Forrest, CA, the infanticide of John Doe at Christ Hospital in Oak Lawn, Illinois was in the public eye. Given his stand against the Illinois Born-Alive Infants Protection Act, then Senator Obama's position on when a baby gains Constitutional protection became a question. Pastor Rick Warren asked the Democratic Presidential nominee, "At what point does a baby get human rights in your view?"

Revealing the uncertainty intrinsic to a postmodern worldview, President Obama replied, "Well, I think that whether you are looking at it from a theological perspective or a scientific perspective, answering that question with specificity, you know, is above my pay grade."[26]

Remarkable! Barack Obama, who repeatedly referred to himself as a "Constitutional law professor," was unable to say when a baby gains the right to life, liberty, and the pursuit of happiness as set forth in the *Declaration of Independence, Constitution, and the Bill of Rights.* President Obama campaigned on the promise to reform the U.S. healthcare system. Now Americans must know, is he America's first truly postmodern president? When reforming American healthcare, did he intend to follow Plato or Hippocrates? By selecting Dr. Ezekiel Emanuel as his special advisor on healthcare, I fear what the answer may be. But the story goes on.

President Obama's selection of Dr. Donald Berwick as the new director of the Center for Medicare and Medicaid Services makes the orientation of our President's ethical compass even more concerning. Dr. Berwick remains an outspoken advocate for the British National Health Service and its National Institute for Clinical Effectiveness (NICE). In a 2008 speech Dr. Berwick expressed this admiration for the British system, "I am a romantic about the National Health Service. I love it."[27] Dr. Berwick then spoke about this system of healthcare rationing with glowing admiration; "NICE is not just a national treasure, it is a global treasure."[28]

So what is the National Institute for Clinical Effectiveness (NICE)? NICE forms the rationing body of Britain's National Health Service; it literally puts a value on each year of human life—presently set at $44,305.[29] NICE deems healthcare costs less than this acceptable; healthcare costs surpassing this "Quality Adjusted Life Year" limit are not.

What does this mean for ordinary Americans? Once America adopts a European styled healthcare system, Americans must expect European style outcomes. In Europe, 79% of women diagnosed with breast cancer (and only 77.5% of men diagnosed with prostate cancer) remain alive after five years. Patients in the United States stand a much better chance of surviving. Under the American healthcare system, 91% of women with breast cancer (and 99.3% of men with prostate cancer) remain alive at five year.[30]

5-YEAR CANCER SURVIVAL

	Europe	America
Breast Cancer	79%	90.1%
Prostate Cancer	77.5%	99.3%
	Britain	America
Stomach	16.9%	25%
Colorectal	51.8%	65.5%
Lung	8.4%	15.7%
Soft-tissue	57.5%	65.1%
Skin (melanoma)	84.8%	92.3%

These numbers expose what the words "comparative effectiveness research" and "cost-effective care" mean under a government-run system. As Barbara Wagner found, when faced with massive deficits, the State calculates "cost effectiveness" differently than the patient. The State may consider it more "cost effective" to let a patient die rather than offering the hope of life. Of note, President Obama created the Federal Coordinating Council for Comparative Effectiveness Research four weeks after taking office. He then appointed all 15 members within three days of signing the bill, Dr. Ezekiel

Emanuel being one of them.

History has seen this before and America may see the hidden hand of Plato once again.

Are You an "H" or a "P"?

Physicians did not deliberately navigate away from Hippocrates—they still remember his Oath on becoming physicians—yet Western society circumnavigated the worldview of Hippocrates. Departing the shores of Plato 2,500 years ago, medicine floated blissfully these many years on the gentle and predictable seas of Hippocrates, only to find itself tossed by an ethical chop. Having struck the crosscurrents of Plato once again, America's compass spins uselessly as she struggles to live with two competing worldviews.

As technology, politics, and healthcare policy race forward, our culture exists in a state of unrelenting turmoil. Much of this arises because whether healthcare reform, abortion, euthanasia, or infanticide, each issue requires a fresh decision. Are physicians to abide by their own consciences? Should they detach themselves from conscience and follow directions provided by individual patients? By the medical profession? By society? By the court? These questions remain unanswerable by any authority within the borders of our nation now that America has lost its consensus worldview. So the angst lives on.

Though largely unrecognized, most Americans align their ethical positions with one of two underlying archetypal philosophies. Though teleologically incompatible, the ideals of Hippocrates and Plato have become entwined, blurring *fixed points of reference* for communication and decision-making. America's ethical compass spins uselessly in a world with two magnetic Norths.

Will America find a consensus view as applied to medical ethics and the role of the physician? There are only two choices. Physicians can either return to their Hippocratic roots and remain devoted to serve the individual patient's well-being, or they will follow Plato and become servants of the State. The archives of history tell us there is no third alternative.

Each American must ask, "Where does my compass point? Where is true North? What future do I want for American healthcare?" Hopefully, recognizing this basic polarization of thought will encourage clear dialogue as America contemplates the future of American healthcare. Otherwise, it may be that for a time, even as in early Greece, this nation will have two "medicines." Or worse, Washington may take us down a road that inevitably ends in the world of Plato.

America just crossed the threshold of fundamental healthcare reform. But the question still remains: Are you an "H" or a "P"?

HIPPOCRATES	PLATO
• Accepted the concept of a fixed Truth	• Rejected the concept of a fixed Truth
• Believed in the intrinsic value of human life	• Believed the philosopher king should determine the value of human life
• Thought medicine should serve well-being of the patient	• Thought medicine should serve welfare of the State
• Rejected infanticide and euthanasia	• Accepted infanticide and euthanasia
• The common man could appeal to a higher moral code	• The State could do as it wished

Notes

1   I want to give the program director of my medical residency, Dr. Henry Weil, a special note of thanks for helping refine and express many ideas found in this chapter. Without his input and skill, this chapter would never have found its present form.

2   Nancy Pelosi, Remarks at the 2010 Legislative Conference for the National Association of Counties, March 9, 2010.

3   Plato, *The Republic*, translated by Benjamin Jowett, (New York: Barnes & Noble Books, 1999), p. 93.

4   Tom Beauchamp, James Childress, *Principles of Biomedical Ethics, Third Edition*, (New York: Oxford University Press, 1989).

5   Todd Ackerman, "Texas Doctors Opting Out of Medicare at Alarming Rate," Houston Chronicle, May 17, 2010.

6   Congressional Budget Office Director's Blog, "Preliminary Analysisi of the President's Budget," http://cboblog.cbo.gov/?p=482

7   Jon Ward, "U.S. to owe nearly as much as it produces by 2020, new CBO report shows," The Daily Caller, March 6, 2010. http://dailycaller.com/2010/03/05/u-s-

to-owe-nearly-as-much-as-it-produces-by-2020-new-cbo-report-shows/

8   Connie Hair, "Rep. Ryan Exposes True Health Care Costs as Enacted," Human Events, April 12, 2010. http://www.humanevents.com/article.php?id=36467

9   Congressional Budget Office Summary: The Budget and Economic Outlook Fiscal Years 2011 to 2021, January 26, 2011. http://www.cbo.gov/ftpdocs/120xx/doc12039/SummaryforWeb.pdf

10   Edelstein, pp. 16-19.

11   Ibid., pp. 62-63.

12   Friedrich Nietzsche, *Twilight of the Idols/The AntiChrist*, translated by R. J. Hollingdale, (New York: Penguin Books, 1990), p. 99.

13   Robert Berger, "Nazi Science—The Dauchau Hypothermia Experiments," *The New England Journal of Medicine*, 17 May, 1990, pp. 1435-1440.

14   Benno Muller-Hill, *Murderous Science*, (United States: Cold Spring Harbor Laboratory Press, 1998), pp. 101-102.

15   I had the privilege of dining with Dr. Nigel Cameron, the author of *The New Medicine: Life and Death After Hippocrates*. One of Dr. Cameron's personal friends was associated with this process.

16   Nigel Cameron, *The New Medicine: Life and Death After Hippocrates*, (Wheaton, Illinois: Crossway Books, 1991), pp. 85-88.

17   Roe v. Wade, 410 U.S. at 132.

18   Joseph Dellapenna, "Abortion and the Law: Blackmun's Distortion of the Historical Record," *Abortion and the Constitution: Reversing Roe v. Wade through the Courts*, edited by Horan, Grant, and Cunningham, (Washington, D.C.: Georgetown University Press, 1987), p. 139.

19   Cameron, p. 115.

20   Helga Kuhse, Peter Singer, *Should the Baby Live?*, (Oxford & New York: Oxford University Press, 1985), p. v.

21   Peter Singer, *Rethinking Life and Death—The Collapse of Our Traditional Ethics*, (St. Martin's Griffin: New York 1994), p. 217.

22   Timothy Quill, Diane Meier, Susan Block, Andrew Billings, "The Debate over Physician-Assisted Suicide: Empirical Data and Convergent Views," *Annals of Internal Medicine*, 128(7), 1 April, 1998, pp. 552-558.

23   Diane Meier, et. al., "A National Survey of Physician-Assisted Suicide and Euthanasia in the United States," N Engl J Med 1998;338:1193-1201.

24   Govind Persad, Alan Wertheimer, Ezekiel Emanuel, "Principles for allocation of scarce medical interventions," *The Lancet*, 373:423-31, January 31, 2009.

25   Stephen Williams, "Bioethics in the Shadow of Nietzsche," *Bioethics and the Future of Medicine: A Christian Appraisal*, edited by Kilner, Cameron, Schiedermayer, (Grand Rapids, Michigan: Paternoster Press, 1995), p. 121.

26   Barack Obama, Rick Warren, Presidential Forum at Saddleback Church, Lake

Forest, CA, August 16, 2008.

27   Michael Tanner, "Death Panels Were an Overblown Claim – Until Now," Cato Institute, May 27, 2010. http://www.cato.org/pub_display.php?pub_id=11851

28   Michael Tanner, "Death Panels Were an Overblown Claim – Until Now"

29   Michael Tanner, "Death Panels Were an Overblown Claim – Until Now"

30   Arduino Verdecchia et. al., "Recent Cancer Survival in Europe: a 2000-02 Period Analysis of AUROCARE-4 Data," *The Lancet Oncology*, Vol. 8, September 2007, pp. 784-796.

CHAPTER FOUR

THE BEGINNING OF
THE GREAT DIVIDE

Men who for truth and honor's sake
Stand fast and suffer long.
Brave men who work while others sleep,
Who dare while others fly...
They build a nation's pillars deep
And lift them to the sky.
Ralph Waldo Emerson (1803-1882)

How did America reach a point in her history where a leading bioethicist could seriously endorse infanticide to control healthcare spending? How could a government-run health plan offer an American citizen physician-assisted suicide rather than chemotherapy? Why did a key presidential advisor propose a "Complete Lives System" that explicitly withholds care from the elderly? Why did President Obama choose a man who believes NICE is a "global treasure" to direct Medicare? How could our nation's Supreme Court say the 5th Amendment words "public use" really meant "public benefit" and allow the city of New London to seize Susette Kelo's home?

The answer to each of these questions lies in the expanding power of a postmodern worldview. *Two dominant worldviews struggle for control of America. One empowers and protects the individual; one surrenders power to the State. We the People must understand this battle of worldviews if individual liberty is to survive.*

Multiple questions confront America today: Do *We the People* still accept the fundamental premise of the *Declaration of Independence*? Can we stand with our Founding Fathers and claim that Americans can "assume among the powers of the earth the separate and equal station to which the laws of nature and of nature's God entitle them?" Do *We the People* still "hold these truths to be self-evident, that all men are created equal, that they are endowed by their Creator with certain unalienable rights, that among these are life, liberty, and the pursuit of happiness?" In short, do *We the People* still believe in God?

The next ten chapters demonstrate the fate of individual liberty turns on how *We the People* answer these questions. Do *We the People* believe a fixed Truth and a higher moral code that constrains government? Or do we believe government is free to serve the "greater good" of the society as it sees fit? Does God endow humans with certain unalienable rights as claimed in the *Declaration of Independence*? Or does government grant rights to the oppressed? Is God in fact real making it both rational and necessary to take the "laws of nature and of nature's God" into account? Or was Nietzsche right? Is God dead leaving science as the yardstick of Truth? If the concept of God is irrational, is man left to define "Truth" for himself?

These competing positions not only battle for dominance in American culture, they affect each political and judicial decision made in this nation. *The Battle for America's Soul* explains how nearly every aspect of today's culture war is rooted in these divergent worldviews. This section, *The Culture War*, reveals the powerful forces behind this great divide and their impact on freedom and democracy in the United States. To comprehend the worldviews dividing America today, the reader must understand the history behind the establishment of this great nation.

* * *

The world of ancient Greece, Plato, and Hippocrates lay in the past. Rome had risen to great heights only to fade away. Christendom now held power and the end of the Middle Ages drew near. As the river of human thought thundered down the canyon of the ages, it came upon a man of such weight, of such tremendous influence, that history itself divided. This mountain of a man was Thomas Aquinas (1225 – 1274), the gentle giant from Sicily.

In the wake of Aquinas, thinking in <u>northern Europe</u> flowed into the Reformation, the Rule of Law, and the United States *Declaration of Independence.* Thought in <u>southern Europe</u> flowed into the Renaissance (1300-1600), the Enlightenment (1700-1800), and existentialism (1850-1950). These parallel rivers of thought remained largely separated until the mid-twentieth century. However, they now come crashing back together with enough force to fracture this great nation.

Who was Thomas Aquinas? How did the thinking of this one man trigger a nation's culture war almost seven hundred years later? What ideas could possibly be powerful enough to alter the course of history? To answer these questions one must turn through the pages of the High Middle Ages to find the spark that ignited today's explosive battle over Truth. The importance of this cannot be overstated—*whoever controls the concept of Truth controls culture.*

The single most powerful contribution that Thomas Aquinas made to western civilization was to reintroduce the philosophy of Aristotle. Prior to Aquinas, western culture had lived under Plato's shadow for nearly a millennium. In his search for justice Plato concluded God must be single, uniform, good, unchanging, and eternal. In this sense Plato predicted the God of Christianity as the source of Truth, even though Plato never found Him. Because St. Augustine (354 – 430) leaned heavily on Plato's thinking when addressing the subject of a higher Truth, Plato held a special place within church theology.

However, much like the philosopher king in Plato's *Republic,* the leaders in the Medieval Church grew to rule over the common man with ever-increasing control. In both Plato's ideal republic and the Medieval Church, the elite in both groups retained power by controlling the concept of "Truth." Plato's philosopher kings ruled because they pursued justice. The clergy of the Medieval Church retained power because they controlled the concept of virtue. The ruling class of both groups viewed Truth as a set of ideals that only the elite fully understood. In the minds of these elite, comprehending virtue and societal justice lay beyond reach of the common man.

The single most powerful contribution that Thomas Aquinas made to the history of western civilization was to reintroduce the philosophy of Aristotle.

Thomas Aquinas upset this lopsided balance of power by reintroducing Aristotelian thought to western culture. Aristotle found Truth in what he could see, touch, hold, and examine. Rather than looking to heaven for Truth as did Plato and the Church, Aristotle found Truth beneath his feet. This returned power to the common man.

Using his extraordinary intellect, Aquinas set out to unify the thinking of these two ancient Greeks. On the one hand Aquinas firmly believed in the reality of the Christian God and in the Plato's concept of a higher moral Truth. On the other hand, he also stood with Aristotle and believed Truth could be found by exploring the world around him. For Aquinas, each of these Truths represented a different side of the same coin. A real and orderly God created a real and orderly world; they fit hand-and-glove. To understand one he needed to understand the other. For Aquinas, both faith and science reflected different aspects of the same *One Truth*.

However, by reviving Aristotle's belief that Truth could be found through observation of the natural world, Aquinas set in motion a tsunami of change that has only now fully breached America's shores. Where Aquinas believed in a unified *One Truth* that encompassed both the Christian God and natural science, many who followed him refused to acknowledge the reality of God or the existence a higher moral code. For these individuals Truth lay exclusively under the realm of natural science.

Whether or not a fixed, higher moral code truly exists is the fundamental question that confronts America today. Was Aquinas right? Is there *One Truth* reflected in both a fixed, higher moral code and science? Or were his opponents right? Is Truth found in science alone? Is the concept of God irrational? These competing positions now battle for dominance in American culture.

The "Dumb Ox" that Divided History

Thomas Aquinas (1225-1274) was one of those rare individuals whose footprints remain forever on the path of history. An awkward boy, he stood tall, bulky, and silent leaving him poorly understood by his peers. Out of a sense of pity, a classmate once assisted him with his lessons. Given his humility and reluctance to speak, Thomas simply thanked the well-intended classmate preferring to be thought ignorant rather than arrogant. By concealing his extraordinary mental ability from his schoolmates, the brightest mind of his generation was nicknamed "The Dumb Ox." However, scientist and teacher Albertus Magnus recognized in Thomas what others failed to see, replying, "You call him a Dumb Ox; I tell you this Dumb Ox shall bellow so loud that his bellowings will fill the world."[1]

Thomas Aquinas was destined for greatness. Born into southern Italian nobility, he was the cousin of the Holy Roman Emperor, the nephew of Red Barbarossa, and the cousin of Frederick II. However, he faced one problem: Aquinas felt no desire to pursue the fame and power that came with his family fortunes. He found no pleasure in fighting, fencing, or horseback riding. This lack of interest in power distressed his father, Count Landolf of Aquino. The Count urged Aquinas to consider becoming an influential Abbott within the church. To the Count's disappointment, Aquinas wanted nothing to do with this position and turned away from his family's purple cloth. Aquinas devoted himself to the simple, the poor, and the study of the philosophy. The Count of Aquino never dreamed through this study of philosophy his son would not only shake all of Europe but would one day shape the political fabric of the greatest nation on earth.

Many remember Aquinas as St. Thomas, the quiet, humble Dominican friar. This physical colossus took up almost no space given his inconspicuous silence. He went unnoticed in a room, yet the world was not large enough to contain his thinking. Aquinas served as a hinge upon which the door of history swung. He devoured the work of ancient philosophers. He not only understood the profound influence of Plato over the previous 1200 years, but he recognized the remarkable neglect of Aristotle. When Aquinas attempted to anchor the lofty ideas of Plato to the rational ground of Aristotle he forever altered western civilization.

Prior to Aquinas, much of the thinking throughout Christendom followed in Plato's footsteps. In his *Republic*, Plato established the need for what he called *forms*. Plato believed these *fixed higher ideals* or *universal truths* must exist before virtue or justice could occur. However, Plato lacked their source. The powerful tie between Plato's philosophy and Judeo-Christian thought was that Judeo-Christianity provided a philosophically rational source for

Plato's *forms*. The Judeo-Christian worldview contained an intelligent and knowable God, something Plato knew must exist, but never found. In this sense Judeo-Christian thought fulfilled Plato's philosophy—Plato argued the need for universal truth; Judeo-Christian philosophy supplied the source. For nearly a millennium, Plato's philosophy and Judeo-Christian thought were inseparable.

However, Plato's unreserved devotion to pure intellectual thought proved his weakness. Metaphorically speaking, Plato seemed more interested in a philosophical debate between two heads soaring among the clouds, than for the earthly bodies the two soaring heads had left behind. Plato's intellectual philosopher king ruled his ideal *Republic*; the elite held power, not the common man. Given this, Plato had no difficulty with issues such as infanticide or euthanasia; ruled by the elite, the welfare of the State was supreme and physical bodies were valued less than intellect. In a sense, life and nature were less important than thought."

Before Aquinas, Christendom mirrored Plato's inadequate recognition of the natural world. Byzantine art reflected Christendom's lack of balance, listing heavily toward the mystical. Reviewing art in the Middle Ages, Francis Schaeffer noted:

> Up until this time, man's thought forms had been Byzantine. The heavenly things were all-important, and were so holy that they were not pictured realistically. For instance, Mary and Christ were never portrayed realistically. Only symbols were portrayed... On the other hand, simple nature—trees and mountains—held no interest for the artists... So prior to Thomas Aquinas there was an overwhelming emphasis on the heavenly things, very far off and very holy, pictured only as symbols, with little interest in nature itself. With the coming of Aquinas we have the real birth of the humanistic elements of the Renaissance.[2]

---

* ˙ Christendom's alignment with Plato may come as a surprise given the stark difference between Plato and Hippocrates regarding the value of human life. However, while the value of human life is a foundational concept when discussing bioethics, it is a mere side note in Plato's teachings.

Because of Christendom's profound alignment with Plato's philosophy, change was inevitable with the reintroduction Aristotle.

Aristotle Reborn

Though a student of Plato, Aristotle began his thinking at the opposite end of the spectrum. Rather than searching the heavens for universal truth as Plato did, Aristotle valued what could be seen, touched, tested, and understood. He trusted Reason applied to the world around him. In fact, the basic rules of logic bare his name—Aristotelian logic.

Aquinas endeavored to reconcile the rational principles of Aristotle with the lofty ideals of Plato and the Christian worldview. Some might claim Aquinas subjected Christianity to Aristotle. However, Aquinas used Aristotle to "make Christendom more Christian." How? Aquinas linked the supernatural and the natural; he connected heaven snd earth. Aquinas devoted both his life and his writing to "reconciling religion with reason." Chesterton wrote:

> Simply as one of the facts that bulk big in history, it is true to say that Thomas [Aquinas] was a very great man who reconciled religion with reason, who expanded it towards experimental science, who insisted that the senses were the windows of the soul and that the reason had a divine right to feed upon facts, and that it was the business of the Faith to digest the strong meat of the toughest and most practical of the pagan philosophies... It was the very life of the Thomist teaching that Reason can be trusted...
>
> St. Thomas was becoming more of a Christian, and not merely more of an Aristotelian, when he insisted that God and the image of God had come in contact through matter with a material world. [3]

The phrase "making Christendom more Christian" packs an enormous amount of thought. For Aquinas the basic thesis of Christianity was that a real, personal, and rational God created a real, personal, and rational world. Because humans bore God's image they could communicate. Even more, they could Reason. The fixed point of reference found in Christian philosophy—an omniscient, all-knowing God revealed Truth to man—made true knowledge possible. The idea that God designed man to understand the world in which he lived was so powerful it launched modern science.

However, prior to Aquinas the church had forgotten the power of Reason by devotedly following the lofty footsteps of Plato. Christendom's view of God had grown remote. As Schaeffer noted, "The heavenly things were all-important, and were so holy that they were not pictured realistically.... Only symbols were portrayed." God had become a mystical concept, not a person.

Aquinas advocated the use of Reason to cut through the mystical fog. Reason helped Aquinas better understand the Creator by better understanding creation; Reason tied heaven to earth in a concrete way. By appealing to Aristotle and the power of observation, Aquinas set nature once again in its proper place. In doing so, Aquinas pulled history in his powerful wake; he opened the door for the coming Renaissance.

By appealing to Reason in this fashion, Aquinas loosed two monumental ideas that fractured history. First, he emphasized the importance of the link between the physical, material world of man and the supernatural world of God through the incarnation. Christianity's central thesis is the Creator entered His creation to verbalize Truth and Meaning in a way that humanity could understand. Accepting the incarnation as reality established a rational set of first principles for the Christian worldview. Linking the natural and the supernatural supplied a moral authority that superseded man's opinion. According to Aquinas, this supplied the rational basis for Plato's Universal Truth.

Second, though Aquinas accepted the traditional view that man was flawed morally, he parted company with many in the church when he claimed that man could be sound intellectually—hence his reliance on Reason. *Aquinas gave Reason its proper place in believing that the real world could be accurately seen and understood through the window of the five senses. He believed that to understand*

> Aquinas gave Reason its proper place in believing that the real world could be accurately seen and understood through the window of the five senses. This laid the foundation for modern science.

nature was, at least in part, to understand God. This laid the foundation for modern science.

If a rational God had created a rational universe and communicated Truth about it (first idea), the natural laws that governed the world could be understood through Reason (second idea). Armed with this unified philosophy of *One Truth*, Aquinas opened the door for modern science. In fact, many of the first scientists were Christian. This view of the world—this worldview—not only gave Christians of the early Renaissance a desire to pursue science, it gave them a philosophical base from which to expect science was possible.

However, Aquinas's reliance on Reason had an unintended consequence. Even though thoroughly Christian, Aquinas opened the door for Reason to be severed from the first principles of Christianity. As a Christian Aquinas deeply believed in the reality of God and moral Truth along with the Truth discovered in nature. He combined Plato and Aristotle holding to the concept of One Truth.

Yet, when the reintroduction of Aristotle's philosophy led to the incredible power of scientific observation, for some, scientific Truth become autonomous. For these individuals scientific Truth became the *only* Truth. In fact, because God and moral Truth could not be proven scientifically, under this worldview, these concepts marked the height of irrationality. Stripped of its Christian foundation, *autonomous Reason* declared God and moral Truth irrational.

The stage was now set for tremendous alterations of basic thought. The assumptions behind Reason itself shifted—the philosophy of logic changed. For Aquinas, logic began with the reality of God; for those who held the opposing worldview, logic declared the concepts of God and moral absolutes irrational. The difference between these two worldviews is nothing short of titanic.

Here lies the heart of the conflict in America today. In those who opposed Aquinas we find the first flicker of the worldview that caused Susette Kelo to lose her home after the 2005 Supreme Court ruling of *Kelo v. New London*. Without the concept of a real God there was no longer a logical basis to support the concept of a higher, unchanging, fixed Truth. Without the concept of a higher, fixed Truth, man was free to determine "Truth" on his own. Under a worldview where "Truth" is determined by man, five Supreme Court Justices were free to determine the intent of the U.S. Constitution's Fifth Amendment for themselves.

When discussing Supreme Court appointments, Americans hear the phrases "strict constructionist" and "original intent." This refers to the view that the Constitution remains *strictly* as the Founding Fathers *constructed* it—that the Constitution continues to mean exactly what the Founding Fathers *originally intended* it to mean. In other words, the Truths found in the Constitution are fixed. Under this worldview the words *"public use"* in the Fifth Amendment always mean *public use*, not "public benefit." Under this worldview, the only way to alter the Constitution is through the process of amendment.

However, under a worldview where man determines Truth, whether through science or by some other method, man is free to determine what the Constitution should mean. Under this worldview Supreme Court Justices are free to determine the words "public use" really mean "public benefit." The remainder of this book tells the story of how this transformation of thought took place.

St. Thomas and the Double Minded Man

In the confrontation between Aquinas and Siger of Brabant, a 13th century French philosopher, we see the first shadows of this coming battle of worldviews. Aquinas won his battle to widen the scope of thought within the church, opening it to Aristotle's philosophy and science. Now the inquiring mind could learn from nature and from the ancients, framing these new ideas within the worldview of Christian thought. What so encouraged Aquinas to pursue this was his belief in *One Truth*. He believed nothing could be found in science that conflicted with what was true of God, for creation was a reflection of the Creator.

On the other hand, Siger of Brabant also encouraged scientific pursuit, *but he separated the church from science.* He purported two "truths"—*the "truth" of the natural world as understood by science and the "truth" in the supernatural world as understood by theology.* He thought the church needed to be correct theologically, but it was permissible for the church to be wrong scientifically. In turn, the scientist could think Christianity was nonsense but could believe that Christianity was still meaningful in a spiritual sense. "In other words, Siger of Brabant split the human head in two, like the blow in an old legend of battle; and declared that a man has two minds, with one of which he must entirely believe and with the other may utterly disbelieve."[4]

Aquinas pursued Truth using two paths, science and theology, but he pursued *One Truth*. This unified worldview was the foundation of all his work. He understood that to separate the natural from the supernatural would have devastating consequences. He fought for the proper place of Reason within the church—and won. However, in this fight he saw something that left him silent the remainder of his life.

All his life he had used Aristotle to make Christendom more Christian, to restore nature to its proper place, and to see God more clearly through science and Reason. Now he saw the capacity for others to use his life's accomplishments to destroy that which he loved most; Aristotle, science, and Reason could be used to banish Christ and religion to the realm of non-reason. Chesterton wrote:

> *Aquinas fought for the proper place of Reason within the church—and won. However, in this fight he saw something that left him silent... he saw the capacity for man to use his life's accomplishments to destroy that which he loved most; Aristotle, science, and Reason could be used to banish Christ and religion to the realm of non-reason.*

> ...he had for the first time truly realized that some might really wish Christ to go down before Aristotle. He never recovered from the shock. He won his battle, because he was the best brain of his time, but he could not forget such an inversion of the whole idea and purpose of his life. He was the sort of man who hates hating people. He had not been used to hating even their hateful ideas, beyond a certain point. But in the abyss of anarchy opened by Siger's sophistry of the Double Mind of Man, he had seen the possibility of the perishing of all idea of religion, and even of all idea of truth.[5]

The weight of this realization impacted Aquinas so profoundly that he laid down his pen and turned away from his work as a scholar. When asked by a friend to return to his former life, Aquinas replied, "I can write no more. I have seen things which make all my writings like straw."[6] He had seen correctly.

The Inquisition: Fuel for Centuries of Conflict

The transformation of ideas that took place during the 600 years that followed Thomas Aquinas cannot be understood outside the context of the darkest hours of Christendom. After the Edict of Milan in 313, Christianity took on two forms. The first was a remnant of the early century church devoted to the teachings of Christ, living in simplicity, humility, and love. Many of the Saints inspired those around them.

For example, St. Francis of Assisi (1181-1226) was the opposite of St. Thomas Aquinas in nearly every way. He died when St. Thomas was born, was thin rather than obese, was vibrant rather than ponderous, and loved poetry rather than philosophy. However, he had the same passion to serve others; the humble prayer that bears his name is a reflection of his life:

The Peace Prayer of Saint Francis

O Lord, make me an instrument of your peace!
Where there is hatred, let me sow love.
Where there is injury, pardon.
Where there is discord, harmony.
Where there is doubt, faith.
Where there is despair, hope.
Where there is darkness, light.
Where there is sorrow, joy.

O Divine Master, grant that I may not so much seek
to be consoled as to console;
to be understood as to understand;
to be loved as to love;
for it is in giving that we receive;
it is in pardoning that we are pardoned;
and it is in dying that we are born to Eternal life.[7]

Though born into a family of wealthy Italian merchants, St. Francis felt called to a simple life of service. Much like Thomas Aquinas, St. Francis disappointed his father by trading his family's wealth and prestige for a life of poverty and service. However, by choosing a simple life lived among the people he served, his message of hope and repentance held power. Free from the hypocrisy of the Church, St. Francis endeared himself to the common man.

A second Thomas, Thomas á Kempis (1380-1471), lived a life of humility, love, and devotion. His giftedness as a writer is evidenced by the fact that his book, *The Imitation of Christ*, remains in print today. His words paint an insightful sense of urgency. For example he wrote, "Times of trouble best discover the true worth of a man; they do not weaken him but show his true nature" and "Always remember your end, and that lost time never returns."[8]

The words and lives of these humble and scholarly saints were often lost on the church leaders. During the lifetimes of these men, a second form of Christianity arose. As the official institution of the church steadily grew more influential in state affairs, corruption followed. Some of the highest clergy positioned themselves to become untouchable and exploited their privilege with reckless abandon.

A worldview that does not value human life ends in death, no matter what name it bears. This theme is born out time and again over the course of history.

Men such as Pope Innocent III (1160-1216) gathered tremendous political power by threatening kings and princes with excommunication from the church. During these times, an excommunicated prince or other official could not survive politically. The pope also crowned the king. Should the individual be excommunicated, the pope no longer had the obligation to crown him as to do so would be to crown a heathen. This gave a pope a powerful tool to gain influence.

Pope Alexander VI (1431-1503) undeservedly gained his position through nepotism. He acted as cardinal and archbishop, as well as bishop and abbot, in a long list of monasteries. For each position he was rewarded monetarily—even though it was impossible for him to discharge the duties of each office. The church and the state had become nearly one and the same.

Having more to do with securing power than with following the teachings of Christ, this second form of Christianity became a potent political institution that sometimes ruled with ferocity. The Inquisitions (Roman Inquisition 1231-1350, Spanish Inquisition 1478-1834) produced the bleakest periods of Christianity's history. They resembled the tyranny of Roman rule during the first century far more than they reflected the teachings of Christ. *A worldview that does not value human life ends in death, no matter what name it bears. This theme is born out time and again over the course of history.*

The church authority came to believe they had the divine right, even the obligation, to press Christianity forward by whatever means necessary. As the Church consolidated power over the following centuries, those who did not believe the teachings of the church became enemies of the state. To deal with these heretics, Pope Gregory IX instituted the Roman Inquisition in 1231.

At its heart the inquisitions were about protecting ideas. Manipulating how people thought was essential to retain power, whether competing with the worldviews of paganism, Protestantism, or Islam. Control over ideas even extended to science as late as 1633 when Galileo faced charges of heresy for asserting the earth revolved around the sun rather than the sun around the earth.

Pope Sixtus IV authorized the brutal Spanish Inquisition in 1478. As the grand inquisitor of Spain, Tomás de Torquemada (1420-1498) used torture to gain evidence against the accused. Under his rule, approximately 2,000 people were burned at the stake.

One of the most complete documentations of papal abuse is *Foxe's Book of Martyrs*. The following two excerpts provide a gut-wrenching picture of what transpired at the hand of an unrestrained church. (I have excluded the most graphic illustrations. They are too violent for the purposes of this book.)

> 1) The president of Turin, after giving a large sum for his life, was cruelly beaten with clubs, stripped of his clothes, and hung feet upwards, with his head and breast in the river: before he was dead, they opened his belly, plucked out his entrails, and threw them into the river; and then carried his heart about the city upon a spear.
>
> At Barre great cruelty was used, even to young children,

whom they cut open, pulled out their entrails... Those who had fled to the castle, when they yielded, were almost hanged. Thus they did at the city of Matiscon; counting it sport to cut off their arms and legs and afterward kill them; and for the entertainment of their visitors, they often threw the Protestants from a high bridge into the river, saying, "Did you ever see men leap so well?"

At Penna, after promising them safety, three hundred were inhumanly butchered; and five and forty at Albia, on the Lord's Day. At Nonne, though it yielded on conditions of safeguard, the most horrid spectacles were exhibited. Persons of both sexes and conditions were indiscriminately murdered; the streets ringing with doleful cries, and flowing with blood; and the houses flaming with fire, which the abandoned soldiers had thrown in. One woman, being dragged from her hiding place with her husband, was first abused by the brutal soldiers, and then with a sword which they commanded her to draw, they forced it while in her hands into the bowels of her husband.[9]

2) Esay Garcino, refusing to renounce his religion, was cut into small pieces; the soldiers, in ridicule, saying, they had minced him. A woman, named Armand, had every limb separated from each other, and then the respective parts were hung upon a hedge. Two old women were ripped open, and then left in the fields upon the snow, where they perished; and a very old woman, who was deformed, had her nose and hands cut off, and was left, to bleed to death in that manner.

A great number of men, women, and children, were flung from the rocks, and dashed to pieces. Magdalen Bertino, a Protestant woman of La Torre, was stripped stark naked, her head tied between her legs, and thrown down one of the precipices; and Mary Raymondet, of the same town, had the flesh sliced from her bones until she expired.

Magdalen Pilot, of Vilario, was cut to pieces in the cave of Castolus; Ann Charboniere had one end of a stake thrust up her body; and the other being fixed in the ground, she was left in that manner to perish, and Jacob Perrin the elder, of the church of Vilario, and David, his brother, were flayed alive.

An inhabitant of La Torre, named Giovanni Andrea Michialm, was apprehended, with four of his children, three of them were hacked to pieces before him, the soldiers asking him, at the death of every child, if he would renounce his religion; this he constantly refused. One of the soldiers then took up the last and youngest by the legs, and putting the same question to the father, he replied as before, when the inhuman brute dashed out the child's brains. The father, however, at the same moment started from them, and fled; the soldiers fired after him, but missed him; and he, by the swiftness of his heels, escaped, and hid himself in the Alps.[10]

These are just a few of hundreds of examples of the brutality of these times. *However, I must portray this dark hour of Christendom for one reason: to understand the flow of thought over time.*

Two conditions must be present for any change: ability and desire. The thought forms provided by Thomas Aquinas provided the ability; the savage abuses of the church created the desire. The above documentary undoubtedly created a visceral revulsion in the reader. However, this repugnance and loathing was magnified a thousand-fold for those who watched loved ones burned alive or racked, quartered, and drawn. The intensity of these emotions drove reform in both northern and southern Europe. Even though these reforms embraced completely opposite solutions, they responded to the same events. We must understand the intense repulsion that set these two paths in motion in order to understand the explosive force with which these two rivers of thought now collide.

Throughout history, nearly every revolution was really a counter-revolution, a reaction to the revolution that had most recently taken place.

One cannot understand what is taking place unless one examines what took place before it. Chesterton wrote:

> Men were always rebelling against the last rebels; or even repenting of their last rebellion. This could be seen in the most casual contemporary fashions... The Modern Girl with the lipstick and the cocktail is as much a rebel against the Women's Rights Women of the '80's [1880's], with her stiff stick-up collars and strict teetotalism, as the latter was a rebel against the Early Victorian lady of the languid waltz tunes and the album full of quotations from Byron; or as the last, again, was a rebel against the Puritan mother to whom the waltz was a wild orgy and Byron the Bolshevist of his age. Trace even the Puritan mother back through history and she represents a rebellion against the Cavalier laxity of the English church, which was at first a rebel against the Catholic civilization, which had been a rebel against the Pagan civilization. Nobody but a lunatic could pretend that these things were a progress...[11]

The preceding discussion was not written to diminish the Catholic faith, the Christian faith, or the office of the pope. In fact, the Catholic Church did reform and became a notable force for good. The life and example of Pope John Paul II reflects this. Against tremendous political pressure, he steadfastly stood for the sanctity of human life, including the life of the unborn. He fought along side President Reagan and Margaret Thatcher for the freedom of his native Poland and other eastern block countries. Even his decision to not officially endorse the use of military force in the war on terror reflected his understanding of history. He understood that heads of state must decide when military action is necessary, not the church. The church recognized military force is sometimes necessary, but remembered its own dark hours when it took the power of the sword for itself.

The horrors of the Inquisitions set the necessary backdrop for the next several centuries of thought. Two solutions arose against the savage abuses of the freewheeling, unfettered power of authority of the church. The first limited the power of the church by placing it under the authority of scripture (the Reformation in northern Europe). The second dismantled the church entirely and relegated religion to the realm of non-reason (the Enlightenment of southern Europe). The first subjected those in power to the Universal Truth of the "laws of nature and nature's God." The second freed those in power to create truth and law for themselves.

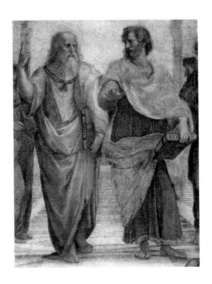

The Parallel Paths of History

The river of human thought thundered uninterrupted down the canyon of the ages until it broke against Thomas Aquinas, a man of such weight, of such tremendous influence, that history itself divided. In the wake of Aquinas, *two parallel worldviews emerged that form the background for America's present cultural divide.* Perhaps these can be most easily understood by looking at the fresco *The School of Athens* painted by Raphael (1483-1520) in 1510.

In the center of the painting Plato and Aristotle walk side-by-side. Plato points upward with his right hand representing his belief that *forms* and ideals came from a supernatural source beyond man. These absolutes and ideals are called *universals*. To Plato's left, Aristotle walks with his right hand extended forward, palm turned downward toward the ground. With this gesture Aristotle emphasizes the visible world of nature. These observable phenomena are called *particulars*.

Thinkers in northern European followed the path forged by Plato. They began with the *universals*, believing the *universals* provided meaning for *particulars*. This theory found unity similar to Aquinas's concept of *One Truth*—a real Creator gave meaning to creation.

Following Aristotle, thinkers in southern European took the opposite approach. They began with the *particulars*, believing the *universals* could be generated independently. This belief followed another principle of Aquinas— reliance on Reason. Note these divergent paths began with entirely opposite assumptions, even though both found roots in Thomas Aquinas.

Even as the Renaissance dawned in southern Europe, the coming of the Reformation rumbled in northern Europe. Each of these two paths must be reviewed in turn.

The Beginnings of Reform—Truth from Above

Following Thomas Aquinas nearly every generation witnessed someone who moved thought and culture toward the rule of law. Each of these thinkers recognized freedom for the common citizen required a fixed law to which the citizen could appeal. Looking at these remarkable individuals one at a time reveals a stunning progression of thought that ends with the United States *Declaration of Independence*.

Born fifty years after the death of Thomas Aquinas, John Wycliff (?1324-1384) was among the first to respond to corruption within the church. After studying natural sciences, mathematics, philosophy and law at Oxford he became a politician, writer, theologian, and scholar of philosophy. In his book *De civili dominio (On Civil Dominion)* Wycliff denounced the commissions, extractions, and squandering of charities by unfit priests. He argued that scripture must be of higher authority than church tradition, the church fathers, and even the pope.

Though thoroughly Catholic, Wycliff is sometimes called "the morning star of the Reformation." In his book *De veritate Sacrae Scripturae (The Truth of Sacred Scripture)*, Wycliff emphasized character, integrity, and dignity and condemned the papacy's lust for power, decadence, and its plunder of the common man to secure personal wealth and luxury. In another book, *De ecclesia (The Church)*, he denounced the extravagance of the church. Infuriated by Wycliff's positions, the papacy burned his writings then, forty-four years after his death, Pope Martin V exhumed Wycliff's bones and reduced them to ashes.

Only a few years later the Bohemian theologian John Hus (?1369-1415) embraced the writings of Wycliff. Convinced that scripture possessed unique authority as the Law of God, Hus believed the writings of church fathers such as Augustine or Aquinas, while useful for doctrine, were subject to the authority of Scripture. In other words, Hus believed those in power were subject to a higher authority to which the common man could appeal. Because he challenged the power structure of his day, the church declared Hus a heretic and launched a crusade against his followers. Using Wycliff's Bible translations as kindling to start the fire, the church burned Hus at the stake in 1415. His death reflected the malice he spent his life fighting.

Hus and Wycliff were among the first tremors of a mounting philosophical earthquake and the aftershocks of their thinking reached as far as the United States' *Declaration of Independence*. The idea that even laymen could challenge church/governmental leadership by appealing to a common, higher law completely inverted the balance of power.

> If anything is true about human nature, it is that power is never threatened without a severe response to protect it.

Hus dreamed of giving the common man access to a Bible written in the common language—an idea the church found imminently threatening. *If anything is true about human nature, it is that power is never threatened without a severe response to protect it.* However, a groundswell mounted that proved unstoppable. A new age of technology leveraged the impact of these few reformers. In 1455, forty years after the execution of Hus, the German inventor Johann Gutenberg became what many consider the most influential man of the last millennium when he built the first printing press. Gutenberg made communication with the public on a mass scale possible. Print changed the world. The first book ever printed with movable type was the Gutenberg Bible, partially fulfilling the dreams of Wycliff and Hus.

Thirty-three years after the printing of the Gutenberg Bible a man destined to take the final step was born. Martin Luther (1483-1546) translated the Bible into common German giving every person access to a source of moral authority higher than the pope. Access to an understandable translation of the Bible, together with the growing concept of *Sola scriptura* (scripture only) removed yet more power from church leadership. This in turn influenced the balance of power in government.

The First Steps Toward Limited Government

The Reformation placed pressure on the Catholic church to reform. Some resisted the threat to their power with Inquisitional violence, but others applied their intellect to the problem at hand. The British theologian and legal philosopher Vicar Richard Hooker (1554-1600) led the way. His major work, *Of the Laws of Ecclesiastical Polity*, was an eight-volume masterpiece. He published the first five volumes in 1590's; others published the last three volumes after his death. Hooker's thinking profoundly influenced American political philosophy in the late 1700's, particularly through the work of John Locke.

That just civil law rested on the laws of nature and the Scriptures framed Hooker's thinking. He wrote:

> And because the point about which we strive is the quality of our laws, our first entrance hereinto cannot better be made than with consideration of the nature of law in general... namely the law whereby the Eternal Himself doth work. Proceeding from hence to the law, first of Nature, then of Scripture, we shall have the easier access unto those things which come after to be debated.[12]

Later Hooker explained:

> For whereas God hath left sundry kinds of laws unto men, and by all those laws the actions of men are in some sort directed; they hold that one only law, the Scripture, must be

the rule to direct all things.[13]

Samuel Rutherford (1600-1661) was born the year Hooker died. His book, *Lex Rex*, proved another hinge upon which the door of history turned. Written in 1644, this astute combination of theology and political science declared *lex rex*, "law is king." Rutherford derived nearly all of his argumentation directly from the Bible on the basis of two primary laws, the "Law of nature" and the "Law of God." *Lex Rex* read like a sermon, which was fitting given that Rutherford was a reverend.

Rutherford's *Lex Rex* profoundly influenced the founding documents of the United States. His work directly shaped the thinking of John Witherspoon (1723-1794), a member of the Continental Congress and a signer of the *Declaration of Independence*. Rutherford's work guided another author, the British philosopher John Locke (1632-1704).[14] The link between *Lex Rex* and our *Declaration of Independence* is unmistakable when the two are placed side by side.

The first two paragraphs on the *Declaration of Independence* read:

> When in the course of human events, it becomes necessary for one people to dissolve the political bands which have connected them with another, and to assume among the powers of the earth the separate and equal station to which the laws of nature and of nature's God entitles them...
>
> We hold these truths to be self-evident, that all men are created equal, that they are endowed by their Creator with certain unalienable rights, that among these are life, liberty and the pursuit of happiness. That to secure these rights, governments are instituted among men, deriving their just powers from the consent of the governed. That whenever any form of government becomes destructive of these ends, it is the right of the people to alter or to abolish it ...[15]

The first paragraph of *Lex Rex* states, "...is warranted by the law of nature, and consequently by a divine law; for who can deny the law of nature to be a divine law?"[16] One also finds "the law of nature cannot be set down in positive covenants, they are presupposed..."[17] "all men be born equally free, as I hope to prove..."[18] "Every man by nature hath immunity and liberty from despotical and hierarchical empire..."[19] "What the king doth as king, he doeth it for the happiness of his people."[20] "The power that the king hath... he hath it from the people who maketh him king..."[21] "therefore upon law-ground they make him a king, and, upon law-grounds and just demerit, they may unmake him again; for what men voluntarily do upon condition, the condition being removed, they may undo again."[22]

To see the nearly verbatim use of Lex Rex in the Declaration of Independence, reread the preceding two paragraphs one line at a time, comparing the corresponding sentences. The fundamental parallels in thought are unmistakable. Rutherford clearly established the authority that preserved the concept of Lex Rex—Law is King: the authority of scipture. To remove scripture from the public sector was to remove the intellectual foundation of *Lex Rex*. To remove the concept of *Lex Rex* was to remove the basis for the Rule of Law. To remove the Rule of Law was to destroy everything our Founding Fathers held dear.

To remove the Rule of Law is to destroy everything our Founding Fathers held dear.

Similarities to the World of Plato and Hippocrates

Here one must step back and pause to understand these truly remarkable events. What transpired between 1225 (the birth of Thomas Aquinas) and 1644 (the publication of *Lex Rex*) was the same battle of Plato and Hippocrates over the source of moral truth, only transferred to a different playing field using different terminology. The parallels are astounding but not at all intuitive.

Acting as an independent political force, the institution of the church had sided with Plato—it both defined moral law for itself and set aside the value of human life. The Inquisitions were church sanctioned horrors, not unlike Plato's treatment of the sick, "...as for the rest, those with a poor physical constitution will be allowed to die, and those with irredeemably rotten minds will be put to death." The reasons for these similar positions differed significantly but much of the underlying philosophy was the same—both the church and Plato believed in an oligarchy, the few ruled the many. The church spoke using words of Christianity but acted with complete autonomy. Law was law unto itself—even as it was for Plato—though both recognized "god" with words.

In a fashion similar to the Pythagoreans, reformers such as Aquinas, Wyclif, Hus, and Rutherford believed Truth and Morality were of divine origin and understood their lives were to be lived accordingly. The Pythagoreans appealed to the Greek gods as their higher authority (for the sanctity of life) to stand against what they thought were abuses of Greek liberalism. Aquinas, Wyclif, Hus, and Rutherford appealed to Christian Scriptures to stand against the abuses of the church. All of these men believed moral law was not determined by human consensus. Only by appealing to a moral authority higher than themselves could they impact their culture. As the reader will discover in the next chapter, this genesis of the Rule of Law is the real foundation of freedom and democracy in the United States.

Notes

1   G. K. Chesterton, *Saint Thomas Aquinas "The Dumb Ox"*, (New York: Doubleday, 1956), p. 71.

2   Francis Schaeffer, *The Complete Works of Francis Schaeffer Volume 1, Escape From Reason*, (Westchester, Illinois: Crossway Books, 1988), p. 210.

3   Ibid., pp. 32-33,36.

4   Chesterton, pp. 92-93.

5   Ibid,. p. 141.

6   Ibid., p. 141.

7   The Peace Prayer of Saint Francis, http://wahiduddin.net/saint_francis_of_assisi. htm, December, 2005.

8   Thomas à Kempis, *The Imitation of Christ*, (New York: Penguin Books, 1988), pp. 45, 66.

9   John Foxe, edited by William Byron Forbush, *Foxe's Book of Martyrs*, (Peabody Massachusetts: Hendrickson Publishers, 2004), pp. 66-67.

10   Ibid., pp. 138-139.

11   Chesterton. pp. 76-77.

12   Barton, p. 220.

13   Ibid,. p. 220.

14   Schaeffer, *Volume 5: How Should We then Live?*, p. 138.

15   United States Declaration of Independence, 4 July, 1776.

16   Samuel Rutherford, *Lex, Rex, The Law and the Prince, Question I*, (Harrisonburg, Virginia: Sprinkle Publications, 1982), p. 1.

17   Ibid., p. 118.

18   Ibid., p. 2.

19   Ibid., p. 53.

20   Ibid., p. 123.

21   Ibid., p. 102.

22   Ibid., p. 126.

CHAPTER FIVE

FINDING TRUTH FOR A NEW WORLD

Give me your tired, your poor,
Your huddled masses yearning to breathe free,
The wretched refuse of your teeming shore.
Send these, the homeless, tempest-tost to me,
I lift my lamp beside the golden door!
Emma Lazarus

Driven by the winds of hope thousands flooded the shores of the new world. By the tens of thousands they clawed dreams from the unforgiving land with ruthless determination. Marked by courage, honor, and fierce independence, they spilled their blood with reckless abandon not only to forge a new life but for the liberty that burned within their souls. Freedom's clarion song had captured their hearts. Who were these people? They were Americans.

Drawing upon the wisdom of the ages America's Founding Fathers fashioned the longest ongoing constitutional-republic in history[1] and out of this grand experiment arose a nation unlike any other the world had known. No other people so willingly sacrificed their sons and daughters for the liberty of others thousands of miles away. Time and again, this is what Americans have done; it is their nature. Freedom flows through their veins. One must

THE BATTLE FOR AMERICA'S SOUL

ask, what heritage moves America's finest to lay down their own lives for the freedom of another?

The birth of a nation is a truly extraordinary event. Only after searching thousands of years of civilization did America's Founding Fathers carefully craft a government. At the Constitutional Convention in 1787 Benjamin Franklin noted, "We have gone back to ancient history for models of government, and examined the different forms of those republics..."[2,3] The result? For the last two centuries the United States has stood as an unparalleled beacon of hope, liberty, and freedom. *"Give me your tired, your poor, your huddled masses yearning to breathe free..."*

> **Did the Founding Fathers believe the American government should determine what is good and right for its citizens or is there a higher law to which our government is bound?**

What were these ideas? Where did they come from? Historian Donald Lutz addressed these questions in a ten-year study. Lutz set out to analyze writings from the founding era of America between the years 1760 and 1805. His goal was to determine whom the Founding Fathers referenced in crafting our nation's constitution. After Lutz culled 3,154 quotations from over 15,000 writings, he tabulated the sources of these quotations. The significance of this study is that it provides an objective measure of the ideas on which America was founded; it supplies an answer to the question, "Did the Founding Fathers believe the American government should determine what is good and right for its citizens or is there a higher law to which our government is bound?"

Lutz found the three men quoted most often were Montesquieu (8.3% of the quotations), Blackstone (7.9%), and Locke (2.9%).[4] Though the impressive political writings of each of these men provide insight into America's founding documents, the primary task here is to understand the worldview these men—the foundation on which they constructed thought. This is the foundation of American liberty.

Locke: The Supremacy of the Laws of Nature and the Laws of God

After Scotland's Samuel Rutherfod published *Lex Rex* in 1644, our story picks up with British philosopher and Oxford scholar John Locke (1632-

1704). Locke was a vital part of England's transition from a government controlled by the king and the church, to a government guided by a balance of power where the voice of the people could be heard.

Perhaps the most important outcome of England's Bloodless Revolution (1688-1689) was the 1689 Bill of Rights. This moved political power from the throne to Parliament. This remarkably peaceful transfer of power was the result of three centuries of effort to wrest absolute power from the elite, reaching back to Britain's John Wyclif (?1324-1384). John Locke lived during these extraordinary times. As part of the Whigs inner circle during the 1680's, Locke was central to the formulation of new political thought intended to end the Catholic monarchy's absolutism. In 1683 he fled to Holland in voluntary exile, returning to Britain in 1690 to publish his two most famous works— *Two Treatises on Government* and *Essay Concerning Human Understanding.*

Locke is sometimes identified as the first thinker of the Enlightenment. For example, at the beginning of the book *The Enlightenment: A Brief History with Documents*, Margaret Jacob makes the statement, "We start with John Locke because he was part of the first stirring of enlightened thought and a major contributor to its success… The Enlightenment began with Locke…"[5] Even though Jacob points out that Locke was a deeply religious man, she nevertheless ties him directly to the Enlightenment. This is actually rather common. In *Total Truth*, Nancy Pearcey groups Locke, Hobbes and Rousseau as they all called for a "social contract" and stressed the importance of the individual.[6] This focus on individual liberty makes sense given their place in history—these men all lived following an age where an autonomous king and church trampled individual rights.

Though Locke did challenge the established church, his worldview was 180° out of phase with later Enlightenment thinkers such as Voltaire and Rousseau. Locke differed from these later thinkers on two basic points. First, Locke believed in the intellectual certainty of God's existence. Second, he used Christian thought as the foundation for civil law. Using the language of Schaeffer, Locke used the *universals* (the law of nature and law of God) to generate the *particulars* (civil law).

In *Essay Concerning Human Understanding,* Locke argued for the certain existence of a powerful, eternal, and all-knowing God that provides the basis for morality:

> **We are capable of knowing certainly that there is a God**... it is evident, that what had its being and beginning from another, must also have all that which is in and belongs to its being from another too. All the powers it has must be owing to and received from the same source. **This eternal source, then, of all being must also be the source and original of all power; and so this eternal Being must be also the most powerful**...
>
> Again, a man finds in himself perception and knowledge. We have then got one step further; and we are certain now that there is not only some being, but some knowing, intelligent being in the world. There was a time, then, when there was no knowing being, and when knowledge began to be; or else there has been also a knowing being from eternity. If it be said, there was a time when no being had any knowledge, when that eternal being was void of all understanding; I reply, that then **it was impossible there should ever have been any knowledge: it [is] impossible that things wholly void of knowledge, and operating blindly, and without any perception, should produce a knowing being**...
>
> **Thus, from the consideration of ourselves, and what we infallibly find in our own constitutions, our reason leads us to the knowledge of this certain and evident truth—That there is an eternal, most powerful, and most knowing Being;** which whether any one will please to call God, it matters not. The thing is evident; and from this idea duly considered, will easily be deduced all those other attributes, which we ought to ascribe to this eternal Being. **If, nevertheless, any one should be found so senselessly arrogant, as to suppose man alone knowing and wise, but yet the product of mere ignorance and chance; and that all the rest of the universe acted only by that blind**

**haphazard; I shall leave with him that very rational and
emphatical rebuke... "What can be more sillily arrogant
and misbecoming, than for a man to think that he has
a mind and understanding in him, but yet in all the
universe beside there is no such thing?" ...From what
has been said, it is plain to me we have a more certain
knowledge of the existence of a God, than of anything
our senses have not immediately discovered to us...**

Though our own being furnishes us, as I have shown,
with an evident and incontestable proof of a Deity; and I
believe nobody can avoid the cogency of it, who will but as
carefully attend to it, as to any other demonstration of so
many parts: yet **this being so fundamental a truth, and of
that consequence, that all religion and genuine morality
depend thereon...**[7]

This passage does not to prove the Christian God exists but it does
demonstrate Locke's worldview. Without question Locke believed God's
existence was "so fundamental a truth, and of that consequence, that all
religion and genuine morality depend thereon..." In a fashion similar to
Thomas Aquinas, Locke's worldview linked the supernatural and the natural
worlds.

Locke believed Reason was fundamental to all knowledge. "Reason must
be our last judge and guide in everything."[8] Taken alone, this sentence could
easily place Locke with the Enlightenment thinkers; but he made a distinction
they did not. Classical Enlightenment thought believed in autonomous
reason—reason alone was the basis of truth. Locke never dispensed with
Reason but asserted that Truth also comes from God. In this sense Locke
was nearly identical to Aquinas, though separated by 400 years. Both men
pursued a unified and single Truth beginning with the certainty of God.
Locke stated:

**Reason is natural revelation, whereby the eternal Father
of light and fountain of all knowledge, communicates to**

**mankind that portion of truth which he has laid within
the reach of their natural faculties: revelation is natural
reason enlarged by a new set of discoveries communicated
by God immediately**; which reason vouches the truth of, by
the testimony and proofs it gives that they come from God.[9]

Revelation vouched for by Reason, Locke accepted as Truth. He further
explained:

> Revelation must be judged of by reason... I do not
> mean that we must consult reason, and examine whether a
> proposition revealed from God can be made out by natural
> principles, and if it cannot, that then we may reject it:
> but consult it we must, and by it examine whether it be
> a revelation from God or no: and if reason finds it to be
> revealed from God, reason then declares for it as much as for
> any other truth, and makes it one of her dictates.[10]

Locke closed his chapter with the conclusion that everything must be
scrutinized against two sources of one Truth: Reason and Scripture.

> If this internal light, or any proposition which under that
> title we take for inspired, be conformable to the principles of
> reason, or to the word of God, which is attested revelation,
> reason warrants it, and we may safely receive it for true, and be
> guided by it in our belief and actions... **[W]e have reason and
> Scripture; unerring rules to know whether it be from God or
> no. Where the truth embraced is consonant to the revelation
> in the written word of God, or the action conformable to the
> dictates of right reason or holy writ, we may be assured that
> we run no risk in entertaining it as such.**[11]

Locke took twenty years to fully develop these concepts, but once
established, he had powerful insight into the foundations of government.

Locke understood the dependence of civil government on Truth revealed through Reason and Scripture. That Locke was influenced by his conclusions about the reality of God is reflected by the fact he referenced the Bible 1,349 times in his *First Treatise on Government* and another 157 times in the *Second Treatise on Government*.[12] This direct linking of Scripture to political theory is remarkably similar to Reverend Samuel Rutherford's *Lex Rex*.

Drawing from this philosophical base, Locke argued for liberty and equality based upon natural rights, i.e. inalienable rights. He supported the private ownership of land and maintained the state should not be able to usurp it—the principle rejected in the recent Supreme Court ruling of *Kelo v. New London*. He called for limited government believing the people retained supreme power, only lending the authority needed for security and social order—a principle expressly violated by the State of Oregon in its treatment of Barbara Wagner.

Locke believed that freedom for every citizen occurred within the bounds of moral and social law. In his social contract he gave both citizens and government responsibility. *Salus populi suprema lex*, "the safety of the people is the supreme law," was the primary responsibility of the government. To obey civil law and live in an orderly fashion was the responsibility of the people. He advocated religious tolerance where people worshiped of their own volition, not from compulsion.

Though Protestant, Locke drew from the Catholic writings of Vicar Richard Hooker. In *Two Treatises on Government* he references Hooker thirteen times, sometimes calling him "the judicious Hooker." A theme that recurs in the works of both these men was also a prominent, recurring thesis in Rutherford's *Lex Rex*. The foundational concepts of the "law of nature" and "the law of God" closely linked the thinking of all three men. These two immutable laws framed the rest of their political and legal thinking. For example Locke states:

> Drawing from this base, Locke argued for liberty and equality based upon natural rights, i.e. inalienable rights. He supported the private ownership of land and maintained the state should not be able to usurp it—the principle rejected in the recent Supreme Court ruling of Kelo v. New London.

> [T]he law of nature stands as an eternal rule to all men, legislators as well as others. The rules that they make for other men's actions, must, as well as their own and other men's actions, be conformable to the law of nature, i.e. to the will of God...[13]

In the following paragraph he footnotes Hooker:

> Human laws are measures in respect of men whose actions they must direct, howbeit **such measures... have also their higher rules to be measured by, which rules are two, the law of God, and the law of nature; so that laws human must be made according to the general laws of nature, and without contradiction to any positive law of scripture, otherwise they are ill made.**[14]

Remarkably, some themes are replayed time and again throughout history. Much like Hippocrates used Pythagorean philosophy to protect the individual patient against the State in medicine, Locke used Christian philosophy to protect the individual citizen against the will of the State. Both Hippocrates and Locke knew the common man needed a fixed point of reference to protect individual liberty.

Montesquieu: Christianity Provides the Necessary Fixed Point of Reference for Sociey

In Donald Lutz's study, Frenchman Baron Charles Secondat de Montesquieu (1689-1755) was referenced more than any other single writer accounting for 8.3% of the quotations used by our Founding Fathers. Why was he quoted so often? Because he addressed two of the issues so vital to our nations political structure—he expanded the idea of separation of powers and the rule of law.

An avid student of history, Montesquieu observed three types of government: despotism ruled by a dictator, a monarchy ruled by a king or queen, and a republic ruled by an elected leader. He strongly favored the republic where the people ultimately held power. Democratically elected leaders were further restrained by both the rule of law and the balance of power among those elected.

Montesquieu proposed three branches of government as America has today with only slight modification. The king enforced law (executive branch), the parliament made law (legislative branch), and the courts interpreted law (judicial branch). He knew it was essential to balance power among these three branches. So foundational was this concept that he wrote, "When the legislative and executive powers are united in the same person, or in the same body of magistrates, there can be no liberty."[15]

Montesquieu's worldview does not fall cleanly into Schaeffer's paradigm of northern European and southern European thought. Montesquieu attacked the Catholic Church in a fashion similar to his southern European contemporaries, and like his fellow Enlightenment French philosophers, he was not devoutly religious. These perspectives stood in contrast to the northern European thinkers Wycliff, Huss, Luther, Hooker, Rutherford, and Locke. These men believed the existence of a real God provided a fixed moral base for human law, civil government, and inalienable rights. Certain things were right and true because they were right and true. Montesquieu did not share these passions. To Montesquieu, Christianity seemed more of a necessary convention.

An avid student of history, Montesquieu observed three types of government: despotism ruled by a dictator, a monarchy ruled by a king or queen, and a republic ruled by an elected leader. He strongly favored the republic where the people ultimately held power. Democratically elected leaders were further restrained by both the rule of law and the balance of power among those elected.

However, rather than seeking to dismantle Christian thought, as many of his Enlightenment colleagues did, Montesquieu embraced it. In doing so he blended the worldviews of both northern and southern Europe. In his book *The Spirit of Laws* (1748) he wrote, "The Christian religion, which ordains that men should love each other, would, without doubt, have every nation blest with the best civil, the best political laws; because these, next to this religion, are the greatest good that men can give and receive."[16]

When speaking of the foundation of civil law, Montesquieu believed there must be a fixed, unmovable base for a society to survive. Religion, *i.e.*

THE BATTLE FOR AMERICA'S SOUL

Christianity (as just noted), was that base.

> *Of Laws divine and human.* We ought not to decide by divine laws what should be decided by human laws; nor determine by human what should be determined by divine laws.
>
> These two sorts of laws differ in their origin, in their object, and in their nature.
>
> It is universally acknowledged, that human laws are, in their own nature, different from those of religion; this is an important principle: but this principle is itself subject to others, which must be inquired into.
>
> **It is in the nature of human laws to... vary in proportion as the will of man changes; on the contrary, by the nature of the laws of religion, they are never to vary. Human laws appoint for some good; those of religion for the best**: good may have another object, because there are many kinds of good; but the best is but one; it cannot therefore change. We may alter laws, because they are reputed no more than good; but the institutions of religion are always supposed to be the best.
>
> There are kingdoms in which the laws are of no value as they depend only on the capricious and fickle humour of the sovereign. If in these kingdoms the laws of religion were of the same nature as the human institutions, the laws of religion too would be of no value. **It is however, necessary to the society that it should have something fixed; and it is religion that has this stability.**[17]

Blackstone: Human Law Depends Upon the Law of Nature and Scripture

Sir William Blackstone (1723-1780), an English law professor and judge, contributed 7.9% of the quotes used by the Founding Fathers. He died after the *Declaration of Independence* was written, completing the line of Reason from Thomas Aquinas to our nation's Founding Fathers.

Blackstone accomplished the remarkable feat of condensing English common law into a clear, cogent four-volume set published as the *Commentaries on the Laws of England* (1765-1769). This timing optimized the impact on the development of the United States' civil law. Seven years after the last volume was published, the colonies began their road to independence. Blackstone's *Commentaries* became definitive because it was the clearest, most concise legal text in print. Thomas Jefferson once quipped that American lawyers used Blackstone's *Commentaries* with the same dedication and reverence that Muslims used the Koran.[18,19] This remained the case until former Chief Justice James Kent published his own four volume *Commentaries on American Law* (1826-1830) sixty years later.

What did Blackstone consider to be the foundation of law? Sounding much like Locke's *Essay Concerning Human Understanding* (see above), Blackstone's *Commentaries* gives us a precise answer:

> **Man, considered as a creature, must necessarily be subject to the laws of his creator, for he is entirely a dependent being**... And consequently as man depends absolutely upon his maker for every thing, it is necessary that he should in all points conform to his maker's will.
>
> **This will of his maker is called the law of nature**... so, when he created man, and endued him with freewill to conduct himself in all parts of life, he laid down certain immutable laws of human nature, whereby that freewill is in some degree regulated and restrained...
>
> Considering the creator only as a being of infinite power, he was able unquestionably to have prescribed whatever laws he pleased... **These are the eternal, immutable laws of good and evil...**
>
> **This law of nature, being coeval [coexistent] with mankind and dictated by God himself, is of course superior in obligation to any other. It is binding over all**

the globe in all countries, and at all times; no human laws are of any validity, if contrary to this: and such of them as are valid derive all their force, and all their authority, mediately or immediately, from this original…

…The doctrines thus delivered we call the revealed or divine law, and they are to be found only in the holy scriptures. These precepts, when revealed, are found upon comparison to be really a part of the original law of nature…

Upon these two foundations, the law of nature and the law of revelation, depend all human laws; that is to say, no human laws should be suffered to contradict these. [20]

The Thread that Ties Aquinas to America's *Declaration of Independence*

A line of Reason can be clearly traced from Thomas Aquinas to America's *Declaration of Independence.* The thread that links the thinking of Aquinas, Wycliff, Huss, Luther, Hooker, Rutherford, Locke, Montesquieu, and Blackstone is their worldview, their belief in the necessity of a *fixed moral base.* Judeo-Christian thought provided this. Time and again these men used the phrases "the laws of nature" and "the laws of God" maintaining that civil laws were subject to these. With the possible exception of Montesquieu, they all believed in the reality of God and that scripture revealed a fixed moral code. Recall that:

Hooker maintained,

Human laws… also [have] higher rules to be measured by, which rules are two, the law of God, and the law of nature; so that laws human must be made according to the general laws of nature, and without contradiction to any positive law of scripture, otherwise they are ill made.

Rutherford began *Lex Rex,*

> The question is either of government in general, or of particular species of government, such as government by one only, called monarchy, the government by some chief leading men, named aristocracy, the government of the people, going under the name democracy... What is warranted by the direction of nature's light is warranted by the law of nature, and consequently by a divine law; for who can deny the law of nature to be a divine law? [The] power of government in general must be from God... All civil power is immediately from God in its root.[21]

Locke noted,

> [T]he law of nature stands as an eternal rule to all men, legislators as well as others. The rules that they make for other men's actions, must, as well as their own and other men's actions, be conformable to the law of nature, i.e. to the will of God.
>
> [Y]et this being so fundamental a truth, and of that consequence, that all religion and genuine morality depend thereon.

A line of Reason can be clearly traced from Thomas Aquinas to America's Declaration of Independence. The thread that links the thinking of Aquinas, Wycliff, Huss, Luther, Hooker, Rutherford, Locke, Montesquieu, and Blackstone is their worldview, their belief in the necessity of a fixed moral base.

Montesquieu added,

> There are kingdoms in which the laws are of no value as they depend only on the capricious and fickle humour of the sovereign. If in these kingdoms the laws of religion were of the same nature as the human institutions, the laws of religion too would be of no value. It is however, necessary to the society that it should have something fixed; and it is religion that has this stability.

Blackstone summarized,

> Upon these two foundations, the law of nature and the law of revelation, depend all human laws; that is to say, no human laws should be suffered to contradict these.

Finally, our *Declaration of Independence* reads,

> When in the course of human events, it becomes necessary for one people to dissolve the political bands which have connected them with another, and to assume among the powers of the earth the separate and equal station to which the laws of nature and of nature's God entitles them…
>
> We hold these truths to be self-evident, that all men are created equal, that they are endowed by their Creator with certain unalienable rights, that among these are life, liberty and the pursuit of happiness. That to secure these rights, governments are instituted among men, deriving their just powers from the consent of the governed.[22]

Historian Donald Lutz's study of the documents the Founding Fathers used to create the social/political framework of our new nation found one other source that accounted for 34% of the direct quotations.[23] This source was quoted over four times more frequently than either Montesquieu or Blackstone and nearly twelve times more frequently that Locke. What was this source? The Bible. This overwhelmingly demonstrates the Judeo-Christian underpinnings of America.

The Founders of our nation knew that it was necessary to have a fixed point from which all else could be judged. As Jean Paul Sartre observed, *no finite point has any meaning unless it has an infinite point of reference.* Judeo-Christian thought provided this infinite point of reference. This understanding of reality reaches back to the *one Truth* of Thomas Aquinas. A real and personal God created a real and personal world to be governed by a fixed moral code.

The Dissolving Age of Hegemony

Volumes could be written about the influence of Christianity in early American history. However, the story of interest in this book lies elsewhere. Others have written about early American history; we seek to understand the present battle for America's soul. To understand this we must turn to the story of the American university because it was in the world of academia that Christians gave away their strategic advantage. The title of a book by George Marsden puts it so aptly, *The Soul of the American University: From Protestant Establishment to Established Nonbelief.*

What caused this fatal oversight? Nineteenth century Christians did not understand the power of a worldview. It was nearly 150 years before conservatives mounted an intelligent rebuttal in an attempt to reclaim it. By then, however, American culture had all but expelled conservative thought from public education.

Public education speaks volumes about culture. Education both shapes and is shaped by the governing public ethos. Educational institutions give culture its worldview, and the dominant worldview determines how every other debate is framed. Whoever controls education controls culture.

Ten years after the Mayflower landed, the Puritan exodus from England began in earnest. The Pilgrims brought Reformation ideals with them including an emphasis on education. In fact men such as Martin Luther were among the most educated men of Old Europe and wore a scholar's gown for preaching. When the Puritans settled in the northeast, Boston had one of the highest concentrations of university-educated men in the world.[24] Higher education naturally became one of the pillars on which our country was built. Against this backdrop, it is no surprise that New England rose to dominate America's higher education for the next three centuries.

Only sixteen years after the signing of the Mayflower Compact, Harvard was established in 1636. This preceded Charles Darwin and the rise of scientific supremacy in education by more than two hundred years. In this era, authority lay in the mastery of languages, not the sciences. The intimate knowledge of ancient texts, including Scripture, was the basis on which the authority of the Inquisitional Church could be challenged—the approach of Scottish theologian Samuel Rutherford (Rutherford published *Lex Rex* eight years after the establishment of Harvard). Clergy significantly influenced the birth of our nation by helping establish the first colleges and universities; this linked public education closely to the church in the founding era.

Notre Dame history professor, George Marsden, explores this connection in his book, *The Soul of the American University—From Protestant Establishment to Established Nonbelief*. He notes, "For the first three centuries of American higher education, the dominant view was that such dual functions [serving both church and state] were easily compatible." He goes on to say:

> The primary purpose of Harvard College was, accordingly, the training of clergy.
>
> Nonetheless, as the sacred and the secular were not sharply differentiated... the Puritans had no difficulty in maintaining the traditional dual purposes of Christendom's university, serving the temporal as well as the civil order.... Just over half (52 percent) of Harvard graduates in the seventeenth century became clergy.[25]

The central role of the clergy in community life appeared again in the Revolutionary era; many of the militia leaders were clergy. These men of education, conviction, and vision molded the New World they found themselves in. For example, the famous fire and brimstone evangelist, Jonathan Edwards, entered Yale at age thirteen and graduated four years later at the head of his class. He went on to become the president of Princeton University in 1757.

Christianity dominated higher education. It has been said that 123 of the first 126 colleges in the United States were of Christian origin.[26] The Congregationalists founded Yale in 1701, finally receiving its charter in 1745. The Anglicans opened William and Mary in 1707. Princeton was founded in 1746 by the Presbyterians, Brown in 1764 by the Baptists. The Dutch Reformed established Rutgers in 1766 and the Congregationalists started Dartmouth in 1769.

The integration of Christian thought and education reached back into grade school. For example, the Founding Fathers undoubtedly learned to read using the New England Primer. First published in 1690, the New England Primer was by far the most commonly used textbook for the next one hundred years and in fact was used on into the twentieth century. When teaching the alphabet an 1805 copy begins: "A—In Adam's Fall, We sinned all."[27,28] and ends, "Z—Zaccheus he, Did climb the Tree, His Lord to see."[29] The section titled, "*The dutiful child's Promise*," states, "I Will fear God, and honor the King. I will honor my Father and Mother. I will obey Superiors."[30]

The New England Primer also contained the Shorter Catechism asking basic theological questions and providing simple answers. For example, "Q. *WHAT is the chief end of man? A.* Man's chief end is to glorify God, and to enjoy him for ever."[31] "Q. *What doth the preface to the ten commandments teach us. A.* The preface to the ten commandments teacheth us, that because God is the Lord, and our God and Redeemer, therefore we are bound to keep all his commandments."[32]

This sounds much like Hooker, "such measures... have also their higher rules to be measured by, which rules are two, the law of God, and the law of nature; so that laws human must be made according to the general laws of nature, and without contradiction to any positive law of scripture, otherwise they are ill made."

Even Blackstone carried this theme, "Man, considered as a creature, must necessarily be subject to the laws of his creator, for he is entirely a dependent being.... Considering the creator only as a being of infinite power, he was able unquestionably to have prescribed whatever laws he pleased.... These are the eternal, immutable laws of good and evil.... This law of nature, being coeval [coexistent] with mankind and dictated by God himself, is of course superior in obligation to any other. It is binding over all the globe in all countries, and at all times; no human laws are of any validity, if contrary to this..."

Early Christians made a strategic miscalculation when creating the foundations of higher education in America. They did not effectively engage the issue of an increasingly pluralistic society.

This explicitly Christian foundation of education in the New World explains why the men drafting the *Declaration of Independence* and the *United States Constitution* turned to the writings of men such as Rev. Samuel Rutherford for their model. Though there were exceptions such as Thomas

Paine, the vast majority of the Founding Fathers operated within the Christian worldview.

However, because each religious denomination positioned itself against the others to gain influence in the developing nation, they lacked a unified plan to maintain the system they were creating. Sectarian rivalries emerged; alliances formed only to wane. Many of the schools began with specific doctrinal positions loyal to their founder's theology, but as competition for students increased, schools remade themselves to appear "non-sectarian." As the nineteenth century progressed, no school survived in its original form.

Strategic Errors in Early America Education

Early Christians made two strategic miscalculations when creating the foundations of higher education in America. First, they did not effectively engage the issue of an increasingly pluralistic society. It was one thing to have little distinction between education, church, and state when the overwhelming majority of the local culture shared a common worldview. The isolation of the first communities made local consensus relatively easy. Those who held positions of authority in the church were the same people who founded the colleges and created government. Youth were educated within the context the dominant worldview making system self-propagating. However, the growing population and improving communications challenged this age of Christian hegemony.

Not appreciating the coming diversity is understandable given the Christian mandate of the first colleges. The possibility that America would eventually banish Christian thought from college campuses was unthinkable. However, the problem of sectarianism (better understood today as religious denominationalism—Presbyterian v. Episcopalian v. Congregationalist v. Anglican...) foreshadowed the difficulties to come, but the warning was ignored.

Like Harvard, Yale began as a devoutly Christian school. Nearly half of its graduates became Congregationalist clergy and its president, Thomas Clap, held rigidly to his orthodoxy.[33] In Yale's early years, Clap was one of the most sectarian college presidents of the time. Marsden relates an occasion in 1744 when Clap expelled two students—not for committing the unthinkable act of skipping church when home on vacation, but for attending church at a rival denomination.[34] Behaviors such as this roused animosity. If Yale received funding from taxes paid by people outside his denomination (namely the Anglicans in this case), how could Clap maintain such a sectarian position?

Here we must recognize the first rumblings of a storm that would expel Christian thought from the university two hundred years later. The debates between various denominations within the Christian circle would eventually shift to Christian v. non-Christian thought. When this shift took place, Christians were caught flat-footed, giving away the intellectual high ground for the next 150 years.

The feeble response of the growing colleges and new universities to the charges of sectarianism was to promote "non-sectarianism," the first code word for tolerance. Nearly every college was transformed from an explicitly Christian institution whose primary purpose was to teach Christian thought, to a public institution where general Christian moral philosophy was taught as one of many subjects. By not addressing the issue head on, they left the door wide open for non-Christians to use the same argument for driving Christianity itself from the public square. Marsden phrases the dilemma this way:

> How could educators fully serve the church with its particular theological commitments while at the same time serving the whole of society? Closely parallel: how could they be true to the Protestant principle that the Bible alone was the supreme authority yet at the same time gain the respect of the world by being open to the highest other intellectual authorities of the day, whether ancient or modern?[35]

Because these questions were never satisfactorily addressed, the Christian dominance in education was destined to fail. It wasn't until the late twentieth century that Christian thinkers finally responded, but by that time education had been radically altered. The answer lay in understanding the hidden (heuristic) assumptions behind the opposing worldview.

The second strategic error of the Christians in early America was to not appreciate the power of a worldview. They did not grasp the fact that

111

each worldview is based upon heuristic assumptions, and these assumptions determine the logical conclusion of a particular worldview. This was precisely what came to vex Thomas Aquinas so greatly after his confrontation with Siger of Brabant. Aquinas clearly saw the catastrophe of using Reason divorced of the concept of *one truth*, where science and reason no longer began with the assumption of the Christian God. When Darwinian philosophy swept though the scientific world, the underlying assumption suddenly became that God did not exist, that man was the measure of all things.

Sir Isaac Newton (1643-1727) presented an elegant depiction of the physical world, as if it were a large clock governed by laws and formulas. The majesty and power of his thinking spread like fire to other disciplines. Science leapt to the forefront of educational excellence and the Modern Age began in force. With the rise of modernity science defined Truth.

Inspired to pursue similar accomplishments in philosophy and ethics, Christian educators embraced this alteration in thought, oblivious to the consequences of shifting the definition of Truth. Certain that the science would verify their Christian understanding of the universe they forgot the insights of Aquinas. Where mastery of language had once ruled supreme and Scripture was considered the source of moral authority, by the mid-twentieth century Christianity retreated into obsolescence, virtually erased from the American university. In the name of Science, the social sciences had captured her soul. Truth was what could be proven scientifically, even at the level of the social sciences. Faith had no place among the intellectually elite. Once this happened, only time was needed to wash the foundations of freedom away entirely.

Notes

1   Barton, p. 213.

2   James Madison, *The Papers of James Madison*, Henry D. Gilpin, editor (Washington: Langtree and O'Sulivan, 1840), Vol. II, p. 984, 1787.

3   Barton, p. 213.

4   Donald Lutz, *The Origins of American Constitutionalism*, (Baton Rouge: Louisiana State University Press, 1988), p. 143.

5   Margaret Jacob, *The Enlightenment: A Brief History with Documents*, (Boston: Bedford/St. Martin's, 2001), p. vii.

6   Nancy Pearcey, *Total Truth: Liberating Christianity from Its Cultural Captivity*,

(Wheaton, Illinois: Crossway Books, 2004), p. 140.

7   John Locke, *Essay Concerning Human Understanding*, Book IV, Chapter IX, paragraphs 1-7, online text @ http://oregonstate.edu/instruct/phl302/philosophers/locke.html

8   Ibid., Chapter XIX, paragraph 14.

9   Ibid., Chapter XIX, paragraph 4.

10 Ibid., Chapter XIX, paragraph 14.

11 Ibid., Chapter XIX, paragraph 15.

12 Barton, p. 219.

13 John Locke, *Second Treatise of Government*, (Indianapolis Indiana: Hackett Publishing Company, 1980), p. 71.

14 Ibid., John Locke quoting Richard Hooker, p. 71.

15 Charles de Montesquieu, *The Spirit of Laws*, Book XI, Section 6, online text @ www.constitution.org/cm/sol.htm

16 Ibid., Book XXIV, Section 1.

17 Ibid., Book XXVI, Section 2.

18 David Barton, p. 53.

19 Thomas Jefferson, *The Writings of Thomas Jefferson*, Albert Ellery Bergh, editor, (Washington D.C.: The Thomas Jefferson Memorial Association, 1904), Vol. XII, p. 392. to Governor John Tyler on May 26, 1810.

20 William Blackstone, *Commentaries on the Laws of England*, Introduction, Section 2, paragraphs 1-12, online text @ www.lonang.com/exlibris/blackstone/index.html

21 Samuel Rutherford, p. 1.

22 United States Declaration of Independence, 4 July, 1776.

23 Donald Lutz, p. 141.

24 George Marsden, *The Soul of the American University*, (New York: Oxford University Press, 1994), p. 37.

25 Ibid., p. 41.

26 David Limbaugh, *Persecution—How liberals Are Waging War Against Christianity*, (Washington DC: Regnery Publishing, Inc., 2003) p. 11.

27 www.gettysburg.edu/~tshannon/his341/nep1805contents.html

28 New England Primer, 1805, p. 12.

29 Ibid., p. 16.

30 Ibid., p. 16.

31 Ibid., p. 30.

32 Ibid., p. 40.

33 Marsden, p, 54.

34 Ibid., p. 55.

35 Ibid., p. 44.

CHAPTER SIX

SCIENCE AND THE SEARCH FOR TRUTH

Plato is dear to me, but dearer still is truth.
Aristotle (429-347 B.C.)

"Tuwi asonai makaerin! We have been fattening you with friendship for the slaughter!" Terror swept Yae's face as his friends reached into the darkening shadows of the thatched hut for their spears. He rose slowly, heart pounding, eyes scanning the room in search of escape. A barbed spear suddenly burned in his side. As he sank to one knee attempting to pull it free, a blow from a stone axe sent him crashing to the floor where he writhed in pain. Comprehending the situation all too well, Yae's mind raced desperately. His tormentors roared with pleasure as he struggled against the pain, face contorted with fear. Another spear tore into his calf. He glimpsed freedom through a gap in the incomplete flooring—the ground lay fifteen feet below. Hope flashed momentarily as he quickly slipped through a crack, but the spear in his calf caught on the rafters. Suspended up-side-down, he helplessly watched children dash for their small bows and arrows. Soon, he was dead.

In the 1960's, Don Richardson and his wife spent several years living with the Sawi people in New Guinea. His book *Peace Child* details how Yae was befriended, betrayed, murdered, beheaded, and finally eaten by his "friends" from the neighboring tribe.[1] For centuries the Sawi had practiced cannibalism, a ritual developed into an art. To kill someone gathered little admiration, but legends were made from the skilled treachery and deception needed to convince an enemy he had become a trusted friend. For Yae, it took seven months to cultivate his friendship and trust as part of this murderous plan.

Some people respond to this story of cannibalism with fascination, others with repulsion and horror. But the question here is, "Can we say cannibalism is morally wrong?" The possible responses fall into three categories, each corresponding to the Judeo-Christian, the modern, and the postmodern worldviews:

1) Many declare without hesitation "Absolutely! To befriend Yae only to eat him later is unthinkable; without question it is wrong regardless of the culture." People with this perspective base their answer on the concept of a transcendent moral Truth. People with this perspective often cannot understand those who conclude otherwise.

2) Others answer, "Let's study the issue to examine the development and impact of this behavior. We may find that in the past it was actually socially advantageous for the Sawi to engage in cannibalism." This response in based on a modern worldview. Truth is what scientific study proves true—including the "soft" or social sciences.

3) However, a growing number of Americans differ; "I wouldn't do that myself, but I can't say they were morally wrong. Each culture must decide what is right for itself. What is true for me is not necessarily true for them. We shouldn't judge the Sawi." This is the only possible conclusion for the devoted postmodern thinker.

Contemplating the moral acceptability of cannibalism appears extreme, but this serves a purpose. No one has a dog in the fight. Cannibalism does not divide America into impassioned pro and anti-cannibalism factions that clash with visceral intensity. Leaving emotion at the door makes room for rational discussion in an age of charged political and cultural stalemate. Contrasting these responses will help clarify the debate surrounding the question of moral judgment facing America today.

The philosophical path leading to postmodern thought is convoluted. To understand this transformation of Truth one must walk through the logical progression of thought in southern Europe beginning with the early sixteenth century. Traveling down this corridor of time illuminates how one idea sets up the next, forming a chain reaction—a series of falling dominoes.

However, before we can appreciate this series of events we must examine a model that demonstrates *how* societal thought shifts during the Renaissance and Enlightenment. This powerful model enables us to envision the logical conclusions of the two dominant worldviews battling for America's soul. Once this model is understood, the forces driving our present cultural divide will emerge as clearly defined entities.

A Model for Worldviews:
The *Universals* and the *Particulars*

At the foundation of *The Complete Works of Francis A. Schaeffer* rests the paradigm of the *universals* and the *particulars*. The "universals" are the overarching principals that give life meaning; they are concepts that hold true for all of humanity. These concepts included virtue, justice, honor, love, liberty, faithfulness, integrity, mercy, and the intrinsic value of human life. They are derived from the "Laws of nature and nature's God." In short, universals are overarching *ideas and ideals*. (Reminiscent of Plato.)

The "particulars" are the tangible things we can see, touch, and quantify. For example, people, nations, chairs, molecules, companies and specific laws of government are particulars. The particulars are *beings* or *things* that can be identified or demonstrated. (Reminiscent of Aristotle.)

Using this model, only three worldviews are possible. The first begins with a set of preexisting, transcendent universals—these give meaning to the particulars (Judeo-Christian). The second begins with the particulars—from these humans use science to generate their own universals (Modernity). In the third, there is utterly no relationship between the two (Postmodernity). (The following diagrams are modifications of diagrams found throughout Schaeffer's writings. He refers to the top portion, the *universals*, as the "upper story" and the bottom portion, the *particulars*, as the "lower story.")

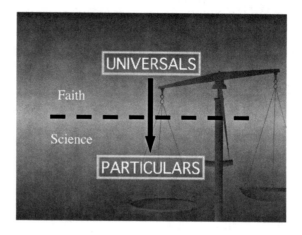

In the first possible worldview, pre-existing universals give meaning to the particulars (the arrow begins in the "upper story" and points downward). For example, because man is created in the image of God (a universal principle), it is wrong to kill and eat your neighbor (a particular law). This worldview begins with the Thomist assumption that God created the observable universe through intelligent design and instilled universal moral principles to guide His creation. This worldview dominated Western culture for centuries. If true, Judeo-Christian thought gives life meaning. It answers the question of *why* mankind exists: a real and personal God created mankind in His own image, infusing humanity with intrinsic value. The above universals (virtue, justice, honor, love, liberty...) are rooted in the "laws of nature and laws of God."

Judeo-Christian thought also provides an epistemological basis for determining morality—the essence of good and evil is defined in the immutable character of a real and personal God as revealed through the Scriptures, not upon human speculation or judicial fiat. If true, the strength of this position is that it supplies a moral standard that rises above any particular individual or elite group, giving form to freedom. This worldview limits how far human behavior can stray.

Empowered by the concept of *Lex Rex* (Law is King), the common citizen gained access to a source of moral authority to confront political institutions, including the papacy. Man was not the measure of all things: a standard existed against which his actions could be weighed, even if he held tremendous political or cultural power. Because Scripture subdued the autonomous power of both king and pope during the Middle Ages it became a foundation of the great American Experiment. For this reason, colleges such as Harvard, Yale, and Princeton emphasized the mastery of language and Scripture up until the late nineteenth century.

British historian Lord Acton (1834-1902) understood the need to restrict governing power. His axiom is now famous: "Power tends to corrupt and absolute power corrupts absolutely." John Adams, our second president, phrased it differently: "The fundamental article of my political creed is that despotism, or unlimited sovereignty, or absolute power, is the same in a majority of a popular assembly, an aristocratic counsel, an oligarchy, and a single emperor."[2]

That human behavior and the behavior of government cannot roam free is a concept running throughout Samuel Rutherford's writings on limited government. Government should be subject not only to the will of the people but also to a fixed moral authority; this is the difference between a pure democracy and a constitutional republic. Rutherford understood "the tyranny of the majority." Winning a majority of the votes does not make a particular position morally right. *To have meaning, every finite point must have an infinite point of reference, even in a democracy.* In *Lex Rex* Rutherford argued this fixed point was Scripture. Unity between the *why* of life (*the universals*) and the *what* of the physical world (*the particulars*) provided this "infinite point of reference" for moral behavior and civil law.

> To have meaning, every finite point must have an infinite point of reference, even in a democracy.

The most significant event of the Renaissance was the alteration of *how* people constructed thought—in other words, during the Renaissance we find a massive transformation in how people searched for meaning and Truth. Using Schaeffer's model, *northern Europe began with the universals in the upper story*—the arrow pointed downward as demonstrated in the diagram above. By the end of the Renaissance, *southern Europe had inverted this paradigm and thought began with the particulars in the lower story.* This is the beginning of modernity—Truth was what could be proven scientifically. Here we find Reason served as the basis for meaning. By the end of the Renaissance the arrow pointed upward.*

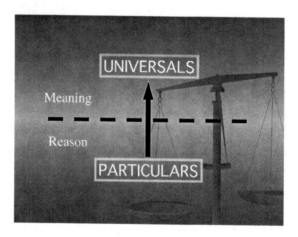

This shift in thought evolved over approximately three centuries affecting various fields of study at different points in time. Art and philosophy were the first to begin thought with the particulars. We first see this in the works of Leonardo da Vinci and Michelangelo at the dawn of the sixteenth century.

Science, on the other hand, remained largely unchanged throughout the Renaissance and well into the Enlightenment. We will examine science next.

---

* (Memory aid) To help remember which is which, northern European thinkers began with universals—thought began in the "upper story" and the arrow points downward (first diagram). Here we found men such as Wyclliff (England), Hus (Czech Republic), Gutenburg (Germany), Luther (Germany), Hooker (England), Rutherford (Scotland), Locke (England), and Blackstone (England).

Southern European thinkers began with the particulars—thought began in the "lower story" and the arrow point upward (second diagram). Here we will discuss thinkers such as Michelangelo (Italy), da Vinci (Italy), Montaigne (France), Descartes (France), Voltaire (France), and Rousseau (France).

By the time we reach thinkers such as Immanuel Kant (Germany) southern European thought has begun to move north. While we find exceptions to this paradigm of northern and southern European thought, it holds true with surprising consistency.

Renaissance Science and the Copernican Revolution: The Upper Story Remains Intact

Following in the footsteps of Thomas Aquinas, science began thought in Schaeffer's "upper story." Early scientists such as Nicolaus Copernicus (1475-1543), Francis Bacon (1561-1626), Galileo Galilei (1564-1642), Johannes Kepler (1571-1630), Sir Isaac Newton (1643-1727), and Michael Faraday (1791-1867) believed the *universals* of Christianity provided a rational basis for the belief that science was possible—a rational God had created an orderly world that could be observed and understood.

Robert Oppenheimer (1904-1967) was the brilliant physicist whose name is now virtually synonymous with the atomic bomb. Though not Christian himself, Oppenheimer believed that the Christian worldview was essential for the birth of modern science.[3] He understood that the Christian philosophical base of the early scientists enabled them to progress as they did. Many contemporary scientific historians shared this view. In fact, in 1958 anthropologist Loren Eiseley wrote this remarkable observation in his book, *Darwin's Century—Evolution and the Men who Discovered it*:

> Although we may recognize the frailties of Christian dogma and deplore the unconscionable persecution of thought which is one of the less appetizing aspects of medieval history, we must also observe that in one of those strange permutations of which history yields occasional rare examples, it is the Christian world which finally gave birth in a clear articulate fashion to the experimental method of science itself.... But perhaps the most curious element of them all is the factor dwelt upon by Whitehead—*the sheer act of faith that the universe possessed order and could be interpreted by rational minds*. For, as Whitehead rightly observes, the philosophy of experimental science was not impressive. It began its discoveries and made use of its method in the faith, not the knowledge, that it was dealing with a rational universe controlled by a Creator who did not act upon whim nor interfere with the forces He had set

in operation. The experimental method succeeded beyond men's wildest dreams but the faith that brought it into being owes something to the Christian conception of the nature of God. It is surely one of the curious paradoxes of history that science, which professionally has little to do with faith, owes its origins to an act of faith that the universe can be rationally interpreted, and that science today is sustained by that assumption.[4] (emphasis not added)

Eiseley asserts the Christian worldview lies at the foundation of the modern scientific method, a position he finds astonishing. "It is surely one of the curious paradoxes of history that science... owes its origins to an act of faith." In the context of contemporary education, the assertion that faith gave rise to modern science is absolutely remarkable. In my fifteen years of formal scientific training I never heard this taught. Yet Eiseley is far from sanguine about the role of religion and appears perplexed by the correlation his research uncovered. The solution for this oxymoronic link between faith and science lies in distinguishing the medieval church as a political force seeking power from the Christian worldview as a philosophy. The two are poles apart.

The philosophical basis leading to modern scientific inquiry is a subject orphaned by public education today. What little is presented is at odds with actual history leading to a significant cultural misunderstanding of the relationship between science and religion. To mention the name of Galileo instantly evokes images of church censorship in the *science v. faith* debate. The two appear mutually exclusive.

While Galileo's theories did upset the conventional wisdom of the time when he challenged Aristotelian philosophy, Galileo's theories were not at odds with faith. In fact it was Galileo's Christian worldview that gave him a reason to believe that man could understand the universe. Like other remarkable scientists of his day, Galileo's faith framed his epistemology. It provided the expectation that scientific knowledge was possible. Harkening back to Aquinas, Galileo believed a rational God created a rational universe and gave man Reason to interpret his universe. Man's Reason was designed to correlate with the physical realties of creation.

Copernicus (1473-1543)

Our story of how worldviews influenced modern scientific inquiry begins with the Polish astronomer Nicolaus Copernicus. The firestorm that bears his name, the Copernican Revolution, began with his book, *On the Revolutions of the Heavenly Bodies*. By no accident his book was published the year he died. This book's hypothesis—the sun, not the earth, was the center of the universe—shook the world. To understand why this assertion was so radical we must return to Aristotle.

The Scholastics, a group of thirteenth and fourteenth century theologians, integrated ancient Greek philosophy with Church theology. Thomas Aquinas was perhaps the greatest member of this group and his effectiveness in reintroducing the thinking of Aristotle cannot be overstated. Giving nature its proper place held enormous power. By the mid-sixteenth century the Scholastics had so woven Aristotle's theories into the fabric of Catholic theology that the Church often interpreted Scripture in light of Aristotle, rather than Aristotle in light of Scripture. Aristotelian philosophy and Church theology were inseparable. This proved significant when Copernicus found Aristotle's science lacking.

In the centuries following Thomas Aquinas the developing medieval worldview was both spectacular and self-contained. Academia rested on philosophical unity. Everything strove to find its proper place in a vast, cosmic symphony—much like the unchanging perfection of Aristotle's eternal heavens.[5] Aristotle believed the sun, moon, planets and stars, all fixed to fifty-five crystalline spheres, slowly traced perfect circular orbits around the earth, returning precisely to where they had begun. The outermost sphere, the Prime Mover, drove the others. Aristotle's Prime Mover fit well with the prevailing Judeo-Christian concept of a heavenly God as the Unmoved Mover.

Everything on Earth strove to find its proper place. Birds sighed for the freedom of flight and stones yearned to fall. From the magnificent to the mundane, from the heights of prestige to the most humble, each part of creation held its station to bring the whole to its perfect destiny. Science worked to understand this synthesis, this "moving image of eternity."[6] Even man was inwardly driven to pursue what was good and righteous, to draw close to God. Yet, on Earth, all was not perfection. Birds tired and ceased to soar. Stones fell only to lie still in the dust. And man sinned awaiting the Church to restore order.

Order lay at the heart of this medieval cosmology. To disrupt it was to disrupt the rules that governed the universe itself. But to understand this intricately designed system was one of the great ends of mankind—to know Aristotle's universe was to know God. This breathed life and meaning into scientific inquiry, yet here was the rub. What would ensue if the unthinkable happened—what would become of this intellectual edifice if science itself proved Aristotle wrong? The Church had chosen poorly. An attack on Aristotle was now seen as an attack on the church.

Aristotle's cosmology had two major difficulties. His model did not explain the variable brilliance of planets. If each planet orbited at a fixed distance from the earth its brightness should never vary. Even more troubling, it did not explain the occasional "retrograde motion" of the planets. Occasionally as a planet swept across the night sky, it would momentarily appear to reverse direction before resuming its initial path. If a planet was fixed to a constantly rotating crystalline sphere, this reversal of direction was impossible.

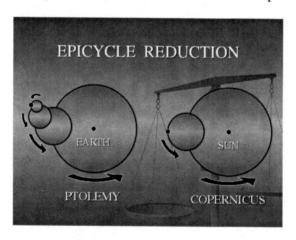

To explain these phenomena, the concept of epicycles was proposed (see graphic). An epicycle is a circular orbit whose center remained fixed in one of Aristotle's spheres, much like a large bearing fixed to the periphery of a wheel. This freed the planet to rotate outside the sphere. Each planet actually traced two circular orbits at the same time, one whose center was a point on Aristotle's sphere and the other the circular path of the sphere itself. Though cumbersome, this provided a solution for the observation of variable brilliance. Now the distance from the earth to the planet could vary as it rotated through its epicycle. It also explained "retrograde motion."

In order to not violate Aristotle's postulate of perfectly circular orbits, by the time of Greek astronomer Ptolemy (85-165 A.D.), the mathematical formulations required to explain planetary motion had become exponentially more complex. Epicycles were added to epicycles in a dizzying array of staggered spheres, each with its center fixed to the sphere beneath it. Copernicus rethought the entire system. Violating Aristotle's first postulate, he placed the sun at the center rather than the Earth but kept the notion of circular orbits. In doing this, Copernicus reduced the number of epicycles from greater than eighty to thirty-four.[7]

The mathematical simplicity of a heliocentric (sun at the center) universe was perhaps the strongest argument at the time that Copernicus was correct. However, violating the laws of Aristotle was not something to be done lightly. Knowing the ramifications of this hypothesis, Copernicus waited until his own death to publish *On the Revolutions of the Heavenly Bodies*.

Though Copernicus saw conflict between his scientific theories and the intellectual/theological dogmas of his day, he did not perceive conflict between science and his faith. His expectation of a regularity, uniformity, and symmetry befitting Creation motivated his scientific inquiry. In *The Soul of Science*, Nancy Pearcey and Marvin Olasky write:

> Copernicus tells us that, in search for a better cosmology than that of Aristotle and Ptolemy, he first went back to the writings of other ancient philosophers. But he uncovered significant disagreement among the ancients regarding the structure of the universe. This inconsistency disturbed him, Copernicus said, for he knew the universe was "wrought for us by a supremely good and orderly Creator." His own scientific work became a quest for a better cosmology—one that would, in the words of theologian Christopher Kaiser, "uphold the regularity, uniformity, and symmetry that

THE BATTLE FOR AMERICA'S SOUL

befitted the work of God."[8]

> [F]or Copernicus "the laws of nature are not intrinsic
> and cannot be deduced *a priori*: rather they are imposed and
> infused by God" and can only be known *a posteriori*, through
> empirical investigation.[9]

Copernicus accepted the reality of God's existence as self-evident and made it his heuristic assumption. This *first principle* gave him the expectation that scientific pursuit was possible, freeing logic and Reason from Aristotle's postulates. When mathematical simplicity (Reason) indicated the sun was the center of the universe, he concluded it must be so. Copernicus differed from the church in that he did not let Aristotle's postulates become orthodoxy; they were merely flawed scientific theory to be rectified. Like Thomas Aquinas, Copernicus believed in *one Truth* allowing scientific inquiry lead where it may. For Copernicus, no *science v. faith* debate existed. Faith pressed him toward better science.

Copernicus began with the universals. The arrow still pointed downward. However, in his use of mathematics we see the first motion toward independent Reason.

Using Schaeffer's paradigm, Copernicus began with the universals—the arrow still pointed downward. However, with Copernicus we see the first motion toward independent Reason. He accepted mathematical reasoning as true in and of itself. Mathematics did not represent total Truth—he believed there was Truth that was not mathematical—but mathematics did represent "pure Reason."

Kepler (1571-1630)

Within thirty years of Copernicus' death came the birth of another inspired astronomer who continued to advance the new scientific revolution. Early in his scientific career Johannes Kepler studied under one of the foremost astronomers of his day, Tycho Brahe. Brahe had compiled the most extensive and precise observations on planetary motion of the time, particularly on the planet Mars. However, Brahe either felt threatened by, did not trust, or was simply jealous of his brilliant young assistant. As a result he only showed

Kepler part of his data.

Kepler was given the task of studying the orbit of Mars, a particularly problematic planet that did not fit the models of the time. Brahe hoped this would keep Kepler occupied while he worked out his own cosmology undisturbed. In a strange twist of fate, the troublesome data given to Kepler was the very data needed to unlock the mystery of planetary motion. Rather than keeping Kepler in obscurity while seeking his own fame, Brahe succeeded in propelling Kepler into scientific history.

Kepler struggled to make sense of the Mars data. He agreed with Copernicus that the sun was the center of the universe. Like Copernicus, Kepler followed Aristotle's notion of circular orbits. The difficulty Kepler faced was an eight-minute difference between the observed orbit of Mars and the calculated orbit based upon a circular orbit. This discrepancy that others discounted plagued Kepler relentlessly. He believed in the precision of creation and in the exactness of geometry. After years of struggle, Kepler finally abandoned Aristotle's second postulate of circular orbits in favor of the ellipse.

Recall Copernicus reduced the number of epicycles from greater than eighty to thirty-four by placing the sun in the center of the solar system. When Kepler combined heliocentrism with elliptical orbits, the need for epicycles vanished altogether. Both the variable brilliance of the stars and their episodic retrograde motion were explained. The mathematical argument for a heliocentric universe with elliptical orbits was now secure and mathematics drew closer to the accepted definition of Truth.

What drove Kepler when others let the discrepancy pass without question? His worldview. Nancy Pearcey and Marvin Olasky describe it this way:

> As with Copernicus, it was Kepler's worldview that drove him to scientific discovery. He described those eight minutes as a "gift of God."[10] He believed a rational God created a precise universe that could be understood by the Reason of man. He wrote, "God, who founded everything in the world according to the norm of quantity, also has endowed man with a mind which can comprehend those norms."[11]

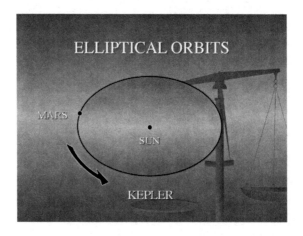

Kepler's worldview was identical to that of Copernicus in that neither saw a conflict between faith and science. Rather, faith made his scientific discovery possible. Scientific thought still began in the "upper story" with Schaeffer's universals.

Galileo (1564-1642)

Galileo Galilei was the first astronomer to use a telescope, giving him insights previously unknown. When studying the sun he noticed blemishes, now know as sunspots, proving the sun was less than perfect. He also provided direct observational evidence the sun rotated, lending credence to the theory of the Earth's diurnal rotation. He discovered the moon was covered with mountains and craters again providing evidence the heavens did not consist of Aristotle's perfect spheres. Galileo also documented the shadow of Venus changed with its orbit in a fashion consistent with the Copernican model. Previously the best arguments for heliocentrism were mathematical models; now Galileo had empirical evidence.

Detecting the moons of Jupiter was one of the most profound observations Galileo made. This demonstrated an orbiting planet would not leave its moon behind. Prior to Galileo, one of the strongest arguments against the Copernican system was the belief that if the Earth orbited the sun everything surrounding it would soon be left behind as it sped through the sky. According to this thinking, a stone tossed straight into the air should land well behind where it was thrown (similar to a ball thrown straight up from a speeding car). With each observation came increasing doubt of Aristotle's authority. Galileo gained confidence the church was intellectually doomed if it continued to wed theology to Aristotelian cosmology.

Modern education often portrays man's myopic desire for self-importance, rather than devotion to Aristotle, as the driving force that secured the Earth's position at the center of the Medieval universe. In a misguided rewriting of history, modern education also depicts challenging this exalted position (the earth's position at the center of the universe) as the reason the church rejected Galileo. Few dogmas of public education are more inaccurate.

The heavens represented perfection, the realm of glory. Medieval theology not only placed the Earth at the center of the universe, but Hades at the center of the Earth. Man resided near hell, hardly a place of honor. When Copernicus placed the Earth in orbit around the sun, this was actually a promotion, not a fall from the seat of honor. As Pearcey and Thaxton note, "Hence the idea that Copernican theory threatened the Christian teaching of human significance is an anachronism. It reads back into history the *angst* of our own age."[12] We must look elsewhere to understand Galileo's conflict with the church.

Central to Aristotle's thinking was the idea of a guiding purpose, or Form. Everything strove to become what it was intended to be. An acorn strove to become at oak, a fetus strove to become an adult, smoke strove to rise into the air, and a rock thrown into the air strove to return to the ground. Everything sought its intended place. The Scholastics reinterpreted Aristotle's Forms in light of God's purposes in nature.[13] In a theological sense, Aristotelian Forms provided a foundation for moral reasoning. Man was designed to strive toward a moral life, fulfilling what he was created to be. Moral behavior was his purpose, his Form. To attack Aristotle was to attack the idea of Forms. To attack Forms was to dismantle the medieval underpinnings for morality. If the basis for moral striving was destroyed, so was the stability of society.

The Reformation brought another perspective, volunteerism. Reformed theologians did not accept Aristotle's Forms. They believed God was sovereign, free to voluntarily create in any way He chose. Rather than being confined to Aristotle's Form of a circular orbit, God was free to let planets follow an elliptical course. Striving to defend itself against the Reformation, the church reaffirmed its allegiance to Aristotelian thought during the Council of Trent (1545-1563) the year before Galileo was born (156).

Galileo's difficulty was that he wished to remain faithful to the church. Like Copernicus and Kepler (though Kepler was Protestant), Galileo's faith gave him the expectation that science was possible. However, his scientific study showed the church's trust in Aristotle was misplaced. Galileo knew that Aristotle's theories would soon be rejected, though the Church clung to them tenaciously.

Yet, it is hard to blame the controlling clergy, the power of Aristotle's thinking was virtually inescapable. In another paradox of history, *so strong was Aristotle's influence at the time, even Galileo himself was unwilling to accept Kepler's theory of elliptical orbits. Alongside the Church, Galileo clung to Aristotle's theory of perfectly circular planetary motion.* What makes this even more remarkable, Kepler was Galileo's friend and colleague. When Kepler sent his data to his friend, because Galileo was unable to escape Aristotle's trappings, Galileo himself could not appreciate what Kepler had discovered.

This paradox of history is so remarkable we must pause to consider its significance. Modern education relentlessly castigates the Christian church for not accepting the science of Galileo; this sets up the apparent conflict of faith vs. reason. Framing the debate in this manner leaves the impression one must choose either choose faith, which makes one an anti-intellectual fool, or one remains committed to intellectual progress and follows scientific advancement. Yet, even Galileo himself, brilliant scientist that he was, fell victim to precisely the same error when he rejected the science of Kepler. So strong was the power of the Aristotelian worldview, Galileo himself could not accept the discovery of his friend. This did not represent a conflict between faith and reason. Fundamentally, it displayed the potentially blinding power of a worldview, even if it was a worldview advanced by Aristotle.

> *In another paradox of history, so strong was Aristotle's influence at the time, even Galileo himself was unwilling to accept Kepler's theory of elliptical orbits. Alongside the Church, Galileo clung to Aristotle's theory of perfectly circular planetary motion.*

Though wrong about the Earth's circular orbit, Galileo did fight for scientific truth the remainder of his life. However, his repeated appeals fell on deaf ears. In the end, the Church never retreated from its Aristotelian ties, largely because of a relatively small number of men were committed Scholastics. Their mission was to protect the Church's ties to Aristotle. In *The Crime of Galileo*, one of the most complete works on the subject, Giorgio de Santillana makes this observation:

> If Galileo had found St. Bonaventure instead of St. Robert Bellarmine still in the seat of theological authority, he [Galileo] might have become a pillar of the Church. But those times were over. Bellarmine was in authority, a masterful Scholastic mind charged with keeping the Church in line with the decisions of the Council of Trent.[14]

At its heart, Galileo's battle was not with faith. He stood with Sir Isaac Newton and many of the other early scientists. Though he did not fully understand it, his battle (even within himself) was with Aristotle. Pearcey and Thaxton succinctly summarize the scientific worldview during the Renaissance:

> The early scientists did not argue that the world was lawfully ordered, and *therefore* there must be a rational God. Instead, they argued that there was a rational God, and *therefore* the world must be lawfully ordered. They had greater confidence in the existence and character of God than in the lawfulness of nature.[15]

Scientific thought during the Renaissance began in Schaeffer's "upper story." The arrow continued to point downward. For science, the universals gave meaning to the observable particulars. However, this would not hold not true for art and philosophy.

Notes

1   Don Richardson, *Peace Child*, (Ventura California: Regal, 1976), pp. 17-40.

2   John Adams, *Correspondence of John Adams and Thomas Jefferson*, 13 November, 1815. *The Oxford Dictionary of Quotations*, (Oxford & New York: Oxford University Press, Revised Fourth Edition, 1996), p. 3.

3   Schaeffer, *Volume 5: He Is There and He Is Not Silent*, p. 328.

4   Loren Eiseley, *Darwin's Century Evolution and the Men Who Discovered It*, (Garden City, New York: Doubleday & Co, 1961), p. 62.

5   Giorgio de Santillana, *The Crime of Galileo*, (Chicago & London: The University if Chicago Press, 1976), pp. 57-59.

6   Ibid., p. 58.

7   Nancy Pearcey, Charles Thaxton, *The Soul of Science: Christian Faith and Natural Philosophy*, (Wheaton, Illinois: Crossway Books, 1994), p. 65.

8   Ibid., p. 25.

9   Ibid., p. 33.

10 Ibid., p. 28.

11 Johannes Kepler, quoted from *The Soul of Science*, p. 130.

12 Ibid., p. 38.

13 Ibid., p. 31.

14 de Santillana, p, 55.

15 Pearcey, Thaxton, p. 27.

CHAPTER SEVEN

THE RENAISSANCE: A TIME OF SHIFTING FOUNDATIONS

Our truth of nowadays is not what is, but what others can be
convinced of; just as we call "money" not only that which is legal,
but also any counterfeit that will pass.

Michel de Montaigne (1533-1592)

The Wexner Center for the Arts in Columbus Ohio represents a fascinating display of postmodern architecture, it stands as a monument to scientific contradiction. A sidewalk appears to end in midair; a "support column" in the main lobby does not touch the ground; stairways lead to nowhere; a portion of the south "wall" is not attached to the building. Architect Peter Eisenman designed the structure so it appeared to operate outside the laws of gravity, as if the building created its own laws of physics. When touring the center, internationally renowned scholar, Ravi Zacharias commented, "I wonder if they used the same techniques when they laid the foundation?"

Even in architecture we find buildings that seemingly yearn for *autonomous freedom*, the same impulse we discovered in chapter one with the Supreme Court decision of *Kelo v. New London*. Given modern science began with the certainty that observation matched reality, how did postmodern architecture end with such illusions? To answer this question we must turn to the art during the Renaissance.

Renaissance Art:
The Particulars Begin to Find Autonomy

Long before Aristotle ran afoul with Galileo and science in the early seventeenth century, Aristotle transformed art. Not long after Thomas Aquinas reintroduced Aristotelian thought in the mid thirteenth century, nature once again had its proper place. Recall that mysticism and imagery ruled the early Middle Ages rather than close observation and authenticity. The Renaissance awakened art to the grand landscape of reality as it was seen, touched, and felt. Schaeffer noted that prior to Aquinas:

> ...man's thought forms had been Byzantine. The heavenly things were all-important, and were so holy that they were not pictured realistically. For instance, Mary and Christ were never portrayed realistically. Only symbols were portrayed... On the other hand, simple nature—trees and mountains—held no interest for the artists... So prior to Thomas Aquinas there was an overwhelming emphasis on the heavenly things, very far off and very holy, pictured only as symbols, with little interest in nature itself. With the coming of Aquinas we have the real birth of the humanistic elements of the Renaissance.[1]

Giotto (1267-1337)

We begin to see how shifting worldviews impacted the progression of art with Giotto di Bondone, one of the first great artists of the Italian Renaissance. The story is told of when Pope Boniface VIII requested a sample of his work. In reply, Giotto painted a perfect circle with a single stroke; this extraordinary talent was recognized immediately. However, Giotto's single greatest accomplishment was to free art from its medieval restraints and balance nature against the divine. A new age had dawned. His depictions of nature contained immediacy and fullness, reflecting life itself. His paintings contained a realism previously unknown—humans were fully human, expressing the breadth of emotion. Though a detailed knowledge of anatomy was over a century away and the technique of perspective had not yet been developed, the rise of the fully human had begun in art.

Renaissance art was not a rebellion against the church. In fact, Aquinas would have applauded Giotto's progress. Nature received its proper place; Aristotle finally tied the lofty ideas of Plato to earth. However, as much as Aquinas would have welcomed the advancement, caution would have checked his soul because the basis of thought was shifting. If one looks closely, the early stages of Humanism are found in the Renaissance.

Individual liberty had long since vanished under the crushing weight of the inquisitional Church. Before the philosophy of Humanism could find autonomy, the human had to be found. Weaving philosophy into its art, the Italian Renaissance powerfully expressed this struggle for autonomy. With stunning mastery the sculptures created during this period reflect the social struggles of the day. Beauty was found once again in the human. We see this in the works of one of its most gifted artists, Michelangelo.

Michelangelo (1475-1564)

Much of what is known about Michelangelo is found in *Lives of the Most Excellent Painters, Sculptors, and Architects*, written by friend and biographer Giorgio Vasari. As a child, Michelangelo's father beat him repeatedly for neglecting academics to follow his love of art. His father wished Michelangelo to be a man of letters, not an artist. Little did he know the world would never forget Michelangelo's artistic genius, lettered or not.

Between 1519 and 1536, Michelangelo sculpted *The Captives*, sometimes referred to as "man tearing himself out of stone." Initially these were considered unfinished works. Now many scholars believe he left them unfinished to make a statement—mankind can set himself free from nature; humanity will overcome. Effort and energy radiate from the sculpture as, muscles straining, head thrown back in pain, man strains to break free from his bondage. Almost as if ensnared in the stone's terrible, suffocating grasp, man fights to break loose to find release from all that binds.

Indeed, man struggled to set himself free. Two years before Michelangelo began these sculptures, Martin Luther nailed the *95 Thesis* to the Castle Church door in Wittenberg. Massive change was in the wind for both northern and southern Europe. Both responded to the same pressures, only in different ways.

The river of human thought rushed on, reshaping culture as it went.

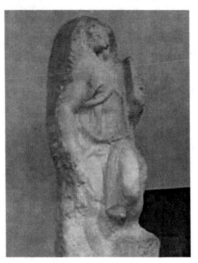

Not far from *The Captives* at the Galleria dell'Accademia in Florence, one can find perhaps the greatest sculpture the world has known, Michelangelo's *David*. Towering 13 ½ feet above his pedestal, *David* portrays man as having attained perfection. Indeed, some would say Michelangelo had done so; the artistic genius emanating from this sculpture is breathtaking. Man had emerged from stone with stunning perfection.

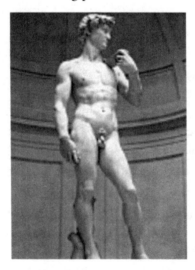

Michelangelo pictures David before his battle with Goliath, face tense, eyes searching for strength and resolve. David is a lithe, athletic, and powerful young man. Michelangelo emphasizes David's personal character traits of cunning, faith, and courage rather than the upcoming battle or its outcome. His David is very human, full of emotion. Nude, sling nearly invisible, David stands alone against the world. This portrayal reflects Michelangelo's patriotism, perfectly fitting the moment of history Florence faced.

Reminiscent of Plato's *polis*, Florence was a city-state. Rather than an oligarchy ruled by Plato's philosopher king, Florence had recently shed the bonds of a local dictatorship to become a republic. This was a moment for freedom and liberty. Facing threat on every side, its citizens were continually on the alert. The Biblical hero David inspired the intrepid citizens of Florence to look within and find the valor and courage required to remain free. Exuding spiritual and personal strength, David prepared to fight for what was just and true against an overpowering foe.

Concerning *David* Vasari wrote:

> without any doubt this figure has put in the shade every other statue, ancient or modern, Greek or Roman... such were the satisfying proportions and beauty of the finished work... To be sure, anyone who has seen Michelangelo's *David* has no need to see anything else by any other sculptor, living or dead.[2]

David, perhaps better than any other sculpture, completes the passage from Byzantine art to the greatest art of the High Renaissance. For centuries, artists failed to depict nature accurately. What Giotto and others started, Michelangelo perfected. In *David*, we find sculpting worthy of a modern anatomy text. Man was portrayed as man in all his glory and strength—the first breath of humanism.

Yet, at this stage of history, humanism remained within the context of religion. (Two hundred years would pass before philosophy explicitly rejected faith, but the process of making man the measure of all things had begun.) When speaking of Michelangelo's contemporary, Leonardo da Vinci,

Renaissance art scholar Giorgio Nicodemi notes:

> [F]or all sixteenth-century humanists, the natural scientists, art, philology, and archaeology were derived from an identification of spirit with life... Spirit was the element which dominated and untied all the phenomena of history. Thus it was possible for Leonardo to unite in art two rather uneasy bedfellows—a fervent religiosity and philosophical speculation....
>
> When trying to express the real value of a work of art... it becomes clear that nature is seen as a repository of that religious truth which allows the mind to function and the hand to obey the dictates of artistic creativity.[3]

Leonardo da Vinci (1452-1519)

Leonardo da Vinci was the consummate Renaissance man. A brilliant artist, accomplished musician, architect, anatomist, botanist, mathematician, and mechanical engineer, da Vinci pushed himself tirelessly. He worked on several projects simultaneously, often leaving them incomplete. The story is told of him leaving a sculpture and walking across town to add two brush strokes to a painting. He was satisfied with nothing less than perfection.

Much of da Vinci's life was spent in pursuit of mathematics and scientific study. His notebooks were filled with sketches of his inventions—most never built. Included were military novelties such as a device for knocking assault ladders from the city wall, flying machines, and even sophisticated waterways to harness a river's power. He never rested, always yearning to understand the world around him.

Da Vinci believed art should imitate nature, but for him there was much more. When composing a portrait, he not only painted a face, he sought to portray the physiological state within, the inner man. Giorgio Nicodemi comments, "Again and again [Leonardo] stressed the necessity for observing not only the resplendent visible surface but also its very viscera."[4] He poured so much of himself into portraying the inner man that Adolfo Venturi describes his art like this:

> [N]o one before him had given such full pictorial life to
> a drawing. As though a dagger, he renders all the deep and
> intimate subtleties of the human body, animates inorganic
> material with living power, unleashes human conflict with
> the fury of a tempest. He undertakes to render the inner life
> of things—of clouds, of rocks, or war horses, of everything in
> the world, in a shower of strokes like lightning bolts or darts
> flashing between lights and shadow.[5]

Da Vinci struggled to capture the soul of man, to lay hold of the essence
of life. Notebooks were filled with sketches in this attempt. Robert Sungenis
notes, "Little known is that da Vinci spent much of his artistic talent drawing
charcoal sketches of the human form in order to capture the 'soul,'—not the
soul in the spiritual sense, rather the inner essence, the universal man."[6] The
Vitruvian Man and the *Last Supper* are timeless masterpieces that reflect his
yearning to discover man's fuller meaning.

Much like Thomas Aquinas, da Vinci sought unity of thought but he began
with the *particulars* (mathematics) rather than the *universals*. Mathematics
slowly overtook him in his pursuit of a unified truth. A correspondence from
a friend written in 1501 noted that da Vinci worked fervently at geometry, so
fervently in fact that "his mathematical experiments have so distracted him
from painting that he can no longer tolerate the brush."[7] But as he aged, da
Vinci recognized that beginning with mathematics, the end was a mechanical
universe. And in a mechanical universe man was a machine; life was devoid
of meaning.

For da Vinci there was always a link between his art and his thought.
Three years before his death he drew a self-portrait. Leopold Mabilleau
vividly describes the weathered, introspective, soul-searching face:

> In sanguine, with an implacable hand, he drew the
> likeness... It is the picture of an old man, a face at once
> terrible and magnificent with the eyes deeply sunken, the

lips tight-drawn and scornful. In the lines we read struggle, pain, and sorrow: a Moses descending from Mount Sinai with empty hands, and without that divine light upon the face that had softened the expression of the prophet.[8]

Despite his genius, in the end he had failed in his quest to generate meaning from mathematics. Schaeffer notes that da Vinci realized that "if man starts with himself alone and logically and rationally moves through mathematics, he never comes to a universal, only particulars and mechanics."[9] Italian philosopher Giovanni Gentile describes it this way:

> Hence the anguish and the innermost tragedy of this universal man, divided between his irreconcilable worlds. Hence the desperate lifelong labor of this implacable self-torturer… leaves in the mind an infinite longing, made up as it were of regret and sadness. It is the longing for a Leonardo different from the Leonardo that he was… It is an anguished longing such as always welled up in Leonardo's heart each time he put down his brush, his charcoal, or his rod, or had to break off setting down his secret thoughts.[10]

Mabilleau describes one of da Vinci's last drawings of himself:

> It is of an old man wrapped in a cape, seated on a tree trunk with his chin resting on a shepherd's crook; he contemplates the whirlpools of the Loire, the river he had dreamed of controlling and turning into a useful tool for mankind. Now he is content merely to watch it in its vain wanderings, as if he were watching the futile meanderings of his own life. In a forlorn, melancholy attitude there is neither anger nor rebellion, only serenity and resignation.[11]

Another 300 years would pass before Kierkegaard solved da Vinci's dilemma of rationally generating universals from particulars—but only by removing the question.

An exploration of other Renaissance artists demonstrates a fascinating progression of the philosophy expressed in art. The universals and the particulars leveled as they search for a state of coequal limbo. The universals retreat but remain intact. The particulars advance but submit to Christian themes. This is seen in Fouquet's painting (?1450) of Mary.

As common during the Renaissance, Fouquet chose a Christian theme. What was unusual was that he chose the king's mistress as his model for Mary. Even more unusual was that he painted her with one breast exposed. Only a short time before, Mary was portrayed as a holy symbol rather than as a real person.[12] The particulars now rivaled the universals. Soon the balance would shift altogether.

Renaissance Philosophy:
The Door to the Enlightenment

During the twilight of the Renaissance, philosophy made the final shift in thought. Where Schaeffer's arrow initially pointed downward in science and was equivocal in art, it now unabashedly points upward. As seen throughout this age, the content and language is unmistakably Christian (*i.e.* Michelangelo's *David*, Fouquet's painting of Mary), but by the end of the Renaissance, the thought form itself had completely reversed.

Montaigne (1533-1592)

As changes of thought and culture in Italy were reflected in the arts, we see the process begin with theology and philosophy in France. Fourteen years after the death of Leonardo da Vinci, French Renaissance thinker Michel de Montaigne was born. Montaigne was a devoted Catholic, well read, well traveled, and reflective. One of his more famous quotations is:

> The value of life lies not in the length of days but in the use you make of them; he has lived for a long time who has little lived. Whether you have lived enough depends not on

the number of your years but on your will.[13]

However, what is of most importance for us is the question he asks in *An Apology for Raymond Sebond* (1576). In this essay Montaigne raises one of the most profound questions that has been asked during the course of human history, "What do I know?" These four words strike to the heart of all Reason. With one simple question, Montaigne put the western civilization's dominant worldview in play. For the first time the possibility arose that *Reason itself— how people thought—might have no fixed point of reference.* This set the stage for the coming Age of Reason, but with Reason free to find its own way without moral boundary.

> Montaigne raised one of the most profound questions that may be asked, "What do I know?" At the very moment the common man in northern Europe gained access to the "laws of nature and laws of God," intellectuals in southern Europe began to question the basis of knowledge itself.

The difference in thought between northern and southern European now emerges more clearly. One year after Montaigne's birth, the German translation of the Bible was printed giving the common man access to a fixed moral authority higher than either king or clergy. At the very moment northern Europe gained access to the "laws of nature and laws of God," intellectuals in southern Europe began to question the basis of knowledge itself.

Montaigne set in motion an uncertainty of knowledge that would amplify over the next four centuries and eventually reverberate throughout western civilization. Before long, Truth vanished into shades of grey.

René Descartes (1596-1650)

Four years after the death of Montaigne, French philosopher René Descartes was born. He stands at another fascinating turning point in history. Like Montaigne, Descartes was devoted to the church, but he separated faith from Reason in a fashion reminiscent of Siger of Brabant. Descartes' philosophy began with "hyperbolic doubt," or more simply phrased, exaggerated doubt. To find Truth, he discarded anything that was not known with absolute certainty. In the end, the certainty of his own existence was the only unquestionable Truth. Descartes concluded that because he could think he must exist. "*Cogito ergo sum*—I think therefore I am."

Using the ability to contemplate his own existence as his starting point, Descartes developed his worldview in the book *Meditations on First Philosophy*, which is actually a series of six essays. In *Meditation 3* he not only argued for the existence of God, he concludes that God must be infinite, good, and perfect. Descartes actually became so well known within the church that some believed he would be a candidate for sainthood. For our purposes though, the fact that he agreed with or was respected by the church is superficial, however fascinating. We seek to understand *how* people think, not *what*. This makes Descartes of interest.

Though Descartes' conclusions with respect to God were congruent with those of Christianity, his logic was radically different. Where thinkers such as Thomas Aquinas believed the *universals* gave meaning to the physical world, Descartes began with only man's knowledge of his own existence and attempted to prove the nature of God. Using Schaeffer's paradigm, Aquinas began thought in the "upper story," the arrow pointed downward. Descartes began thought in the "lower story," the arrow now pointed upwards. Thomas Aquinas and Descartes were polar opposites in terms of *how* they thought, even though both remained devoted to the church.

Humanism was coming of age. In fact, "*Cogito ergo sum*—I think therefore I am" prematurely defined the Enlightenment—the Age of Reason. For Descartes, the certainty of existence itself began with the Reason of man, not the reality of God. Descartes marked the end of an age; he was the last of the optimistic humanists. He believed that mathematics (pure Reason) could be known with absolute certainty and remained optimistic that the *universals* could be found beginning with the *particulars* (the certainty of his own existence). Descartes believed that mathematical analysis would provide a unity of knowledge. However, like Plato and Leonardo da Vinci, this desire went unfulfilled.

The problem of finding universals when beginning with the *particulars* remained unsolved. As Schaeffer states, "Beginning from man alone, Renaissance humanism—and humanism ever since—has found no way to arrive at *universals* or absolutes which give meaning to existence or morals."[14] The arrow in the diagram does not extend completely from the *particulars* to the *universals*; it only reaches half way. The dashed line represents the time during the Renaissance when the two were not yet completely separated. Thinkers continued to hope unity of thought could be found, they hoped the arrow would penetrate through to the "upper story," that ultimate meaning could be generated from the observable particulars alone.

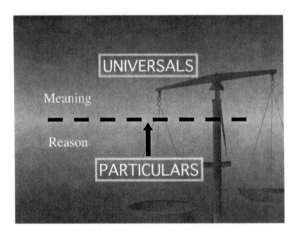

Within 150 years thought had progressed from Michelangelo's *David* portraying the glory of man as man to Descartes basing the certainty of his existence on Reason. Once this point was reached, the Enlightenment was not long in coming, and with it, another fundamental shift in thought.

The primary change during the 200 years prior to Descartes had been to reverse the flow of thought from "universals give meaning to the particulars" to "the particulars can generate universals." During the 200 years following Descartes, philosophers came to believe the *universals* and the *particulars* had no logical relation.

Notes

1   Schaeffer, *Volume 1, Escape From Reason*, p. 210.

2   Howard Hibbard, *Michelangelo, Second edition*, (Boulder Colorado: Westview Press, 1998). P. 59.

3   Giorgio Nicodemi, "The Life and Works of Leonardo," *Leonardo Da Vinci*, (New York: Reynal & Company, 1956), p. 22.

4   Ibid., p. 22.

5   Adolfo Venturi, "The Drawings of Leonardo," *Leonardo Da Vinci*, (New York: Reynal & Company, 1956), p. 91.

6   Robert Sungenis, "Art Through the Ages: Its Philosophical and Theological Meaning," Catholic Apologetics International, www.catholicintl.com, January, 2004.

7   Pietro da Novellara, April 14, 1501, Alessandro Vessosi, *Leonardo da Vinci: The Mind of the Renaissance*, (New York: Harry N. Abrams, Inc, 1997), pp. 88-89.

8   Leoplold Mabilleau, "Leonardo in France," *Leonardo Da Vinci*, (New York: Reynal & Company, 1956), pp. 154-155.

9   Schaeffer, *Volume 1, The God Who is There*, p. 62.

10 Giovanni Gentile, "The Thought of Leonardo," *Leonardo Da Vinci*, (New York: Reynal & Company, 1956), p. 174.

11 Mabileau, p. 156.

12 Schaeffer, *Volume 1, Escape From Reason*, p. 214.

13 Michel de Montaigne, *The Oxford Dictionary of Quotations*, (Oxford & New York: Oxford University Press, Revised Fourth Edition, 1996), p. 480.

14 Schaeffer, *Volume 5: How Should We then Live?*, p. 104.

CHAPTER EIGHT

DEATH OF TRUTH

*Truth is so obscure in these times, and falsehood so established,
that, unless we love the truth, we cannot know it.*

Blaise Pascal (1623-1662)

The day began like any other day for bright-eyed, sandy-haired Jeffrey
Curley. For a ten-year-old boy autumn should be filled with innocence
and wonder, images of leaves scurrying before a cool breeze, or a bike ride
through a park. In fact, the promise of a new bike lured Jeffrey into a car
with two men he considered friends. With that decision, the snapshots of
Jeffrey's life were tragically frozen in time. The new bike never came. Jeffrey
was taken to the Boston Public Library where one of his abductors, Charlie
Jaynes, allegedly accessed the NAMBLA (North American Man-Boy Love
Association) website.

Next, the men drove to a more secluded location and attempted to assault
the fifth grader. Jeffrey resisted. Determined to have their way, they choked
him to death with a gasoline soaked rag. Jaynes then sodomized Jeffrey's dead
body before the men dumped it into the river.

This tragic case drew national attention. The courts found Jeffrey's
abductors guilty of child molestation, kidnapping, and murder. However,
the real legal stir came when Jeffrey's parents filed a $200 million civil suit
against NAMBLA for wrongful death. Investigators had found eight copies
of the NAMBLA *Bulletin* magazines in Jaynes' possession and a handwritten

entry in Jaynes' diary that read, "This was a turning point in discovery of myself... NAMBLA's *Bulletin* helped me become aware of my own sexuality and acceptance of it." The lawsuit cited the *Bulletin*: "Call it love, call it lust, call it whatever you want. We desire sex with boys, and boys, whether society is willing to admit it, desire sex with us."[1]

Framing the case, the family's attorney stated that NAMBLA was:

> ...not just publishing material that says it's OK to have sex with children and advocating changing the law. [It] is actively training their members how to rape children and get away with it. They distribute child pornography and trade live children among NAMBLA members with the purpose of having sex with them.[2]

Enter the American Civil Liberties Union (ACLU); they stepped in to defend NAMBLA's First Amendment right to free speech. In discussing this case in their book, *The ACLU vs America*, Alan Sears and Craig Osten note:

> One of NAMBLA's publications is titled *The Survival Manual: The Man's Guide to Staying Alive in Man-Boy Sexual Relationships*. According to Frisoli [the attorney for Jeffery's parents], "Its chapters explain how to build relationships with children. How to gain the confidence of children's parents. Where to go to have sex with children so as not to get caught." Bill O'Reilly of Fox News added that NAMBLA's Web site "actually posted techniques designed to lure boys into having sex with men and also supplied information on what an adult should do if caught.[3]

The Curley's legal fight continued for eight years until it became apparent they would fail. They dropped their suit against NAMBLA in 2008. Sarah Wunsch, a staff attorney for the ACLU, acknowledged Jaynes belonged to NAMBLA, but insisted there was nothing illegal about the books, magazines, or web site:

There was never any evidence that NAMBLA was connected to the death of Jeffery Curley. It's been our view that for the last eight years, it's been the First Amendment that's been the defendant in this case. In America, there's freedom to publish unpopular ideas, and that's what this case was about.[4]

* * *

For Brittany McComb the day finally arrived; the years of hard work paid off. She nervously approached the microphone, her mind wrestling with what to say. An edited copy of her valedictory address lay open before her, but she wanted to share more. After years of searching, she wanted to explain to the audience what had finally given her inner peace and fulfillment. Her unedited text contained three Bible references, mentioned "God" nine times, and used the phase "the Lord" twice; only once did it reference "Christ."[5,6] However, school officials determined this discussion of faith crossed the line.

After a benign introduction, Brittany's speech rapidly moved toward the personal. She discussed the void she felt even in success saying the emptiness gaped "like a wide open trench when filled with friends, with family, with swimming, with drinking, with shopping, with partying; with anything but God. But His love fits." Cheers rose from the audience when she described God's love. "His love is that something we all desire. It's unprejudiced, it's merciful, it's free, it's real, it's huge, and it's everlasting." She continued, "God's love is so great He gave up His only son..." Her mic went dead.

Buoyed by the growing applause, Brittany's face beamed as she continued without a microphone for more than a minute. Admiring her courage, cheers and applause from the crowded auditorium filled the air. However, three minutes into her talk she knew she could not finish, in spite of the crowd's approval. The energy drained from Brittany's face and the smile left her eyes. Tapping the microphone once last time, Brittany quietly took her seat.[7]

Without saying a word about the highly unusual step of cutting off the microphone of a featured speaker—in the middle of her speech—the school administrator stepped to the podium and simply introduced the next speaker.

The crowd roared its disapproval. Every parent and fellow student knew what just happened. The school had just stripped one of the brightest and hardest working students of her right to free speech—simply because she dared to discus the impact of her faith in public.

Enter the American Civil Liberties Union (ACLU); however, this time they supported the *restriction* of free speech by cutting off Brittany's microphone. Allen Lichtenstein, Nevada's general counsel for the ACLU, noted, "There should be no controversy here. It's important to understand that a student was given a school-sponsored forum and therefore, in essence, it was a school-sponsored speech."[8]

* * *

The debate over the right to speak out in favor of an illegal act remains complex, important, and fascinating. Legal scholars have written volumes on the meaning, context, and intent of the First Amendment. However, our question lies elsewhere. Using the framework of worldviews the next six chapters seek to answer, "Why did the ACLU defend NAMBLA's First Amendment right to advocate the statutory rape of young boys, while simultaneously opposing the First Amendment right of a student to discuss her faith during a valedictory address?" Two simple words encapsulate the answer—*autonomous freedom*.

The concept of *autonomous freedom* is so important that it footnotes every page from here to the end of this book. As we will see, *autonomous freedom* is the tie that binds Peter Singer's proposal of infanticide, the Supreme Court's decision in *Kelo v. New London*, the ACLU's effort to remove Christian symbols across the United States, and even the present-day political hostility that now imperils our nation's future. *Autonomous freedom* is the central thread woven throughout the twisted fabric of America's culture war._

Previous chapters explained how the foundations of cultural thought shifted during the Renaissance. Where universals once gave meaning to the particulars, by the time of Descartes, the arrow reversed direction—he attempted to use particulars to generate universals. Yet Descartes did not really begin with "*Cogito ergo sum*—I think therefore I am" in isolation. He set out knowing what he wanted to prove—he wanted to build an apologetic, an intellectual defense of his Christian faith. He attempted to do this with

Reason alone.

But what would happen if someone used Descartes' method of hyperbolic doubt with a different end in sight? In a sentence, this depicts the Enlightenment—the Age of Reason. Enlightenment thinkers doubted everything not proven by science. However, rather than seeking to prove God's existence, they sought *autonomous freedom*. Strangely enough, it was a gifted Christian physicist that set the stage for this revolution of thought.

The Stars Align: Setting the Stage for Enlightenment

Sir Isaac Newton (1642-1727) belonged to the last of the great Renaissance thinkers and he, perhaps more than any other, readied the world for the Enlightenment. Born eight years before Descartes died, Newton lived during the pivotal pre-Enlightenment years. The elegance and brilliant simplicity of his physics provided the final ingredient needed to transform a world primed for change.

With his three laws of motion, Newton synthesized a universal physics by combining Kepler's laws of planetary motion with Galileo's concept of inertia. He demonstrated the laws governing elliptical orbits in the heavens were the same laws that governed motion on Earth. Newton also developed the mathematical discipline of calculus, greatly expanding the power of applied mathematics. So spectacular were Newton's ideas that the universe began to look like an intricate clock set in motion by God. Everything whirled in perfect order following the precise universal laws of the Creator. Newton's universe was fully as elegant as Aristotle's but accounted for 2,000 years of scientific discovery.

Newton's worldview was nearly identical to that of Copernicus, Kepler, and Galileo. Like Descartes, Newton was a committed Christian who intended his work to be used as an apologetic, a defense of Christianity.[9] Here lies another paradox of history. Aristotle (384-322 BC) had nothing to do with Christian thought, living a full three centuries before the birth of Christ. Yet, following Thomas Aquinas, the Church adopted and strenuously defended Aristotle's flawed cosmology, fantastic as it was, through Christianity's darkest hours. On the other hand, Newton's clarion thought flowed directly from his Christian worldview and was specifically intended to create an apologetic.

Yet, the Church rejected the Copernican Revolution of which Newton was the capstone. Thinkers of the Enlightenment subsequently adopted Newton's theories, using them to cut the Church off at her knees. The irony here is staggering but instructive. Twice the Church did not understand the culture and the times in which she lived. Twice she chose wrongly (first with Aristotle and then again with Newton) and suffered profoundly as a result.

Having examined why the Church followed Aristotle in chapter six, we now must explore the tremendous power pressing southern Europe unavoidably into the Enlightenment as it followed Newton. To do this we must feel the weight of history. Three things were happening simultaneously:

First, the seventeenth century witnessed the Spanish Inquisition. *Foxe's Book of Martyrs* describes the sheer brutality that took place under the authority of the Church. Each victim was someone's parent, spouse, or child—they were real people suffering real torture. As one reads of bodies burning at the stake one can almost feel the smoldering embers of discontent awaiting only a faint breath of oxygen to burst into torrents of revenge. These horrors left an indelible mark not only on the pages of history but also on the souls of men.

> So perfect was Newton's universe that God no longer appeared necessary. For many Enlightenment thinkers, all that was needed to set the universe in motion was an unknown, deistic, Unmoved Mover, leaving man to find the meaning of life on his own.

Second, the world changed following thinkers such as Montaigne and Descartes. Montaigne's query, "What do I know?" called the fundamental assumptions behind western thought into question. Descartes' "hyperbolic doubt" gave philosophers a new way to approach the answer. Prior to these men, societal thought began with the universals as understood by the Church. However, after Descartes, Reason began to find a way on its own. When the embers of discontent flashed into a firestorm of rage, so did the yearning to free Reason from the Church's fetters.

Lastly, with Newton's masterful clocklike universe came a perfect alignment of the stars. When combined with anti-religious sentiment and Descartes' hyperbolic doubt, Newtonian science forever changed the world. So perfect was Newton's universe that God no longer appeared necessary. For many Enlightenment thinkers, all that was needed to set the universe in motion was an unknown, deistic, Unmoved Mover, leaving man to find the meaning of life on his own. This is the story of the Enlightenment—Truth was defined by science and mathematics. For thinkers following this path, the church was relegated to the dustbin of history.

The Enlightenment: Reason Finds Autonomy

If the universe was set in motion by a deistic Unmoved Mover, Montaigne's question, "What do I know?" suddenly took on new significance. Scripture no longer revealed Truth; all fixed points of reference vanished. God was no longer a "Heavenly Father" involved in the daily affairs of man, but an unknowable, distant "Supreme Being." Though God remained the First Cause, He became an uninvolved bystander for the rest of history.

With miracles conceptually impossible (Deism: God set the world in motion but remained uninvolved thereafter), many Biblical stories appeared patently absurd. Christ's virgin birth and his rising from the dead became fairytales created by weak minds needing a crutch to survive. To believe Jonah spent three days in a great fish epitomized naiveté, deserving nothing but disdain. To think God actually sent a great flood after telling Noah to rescue himself and two of every creature in an ark mocked intelligence itself.

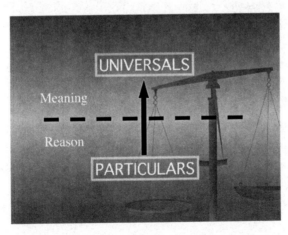

The Church's claim to know "Truth" appeared to be manipulation of emotion at best, coercion of behavior at worst. Changing the assumptions undergirding western thought (whether or not the God of Christianity was real) turned everything up side down. Thomas Aquinas foresaw the significance of this. After his confrontation with Siger of Brabant, without his formulation of one Truth, Aquinas feared religion would soon become one of Reason's principal targets.

For those giving voice to Enlightenment thought during the eighteenth century, this change of worldview emancipated the human consciousness and liberated Reason. Gone were the musty constraints of religious orthodoxy. Gone were the bonds of superstition, ritual, ignorance, and error.

The Age of Reason had dawned. For a brief moment in time, the arrow pierced the barrier granting vindication to the vision of Leonardo da Vinci. Da Vinci devoted his life to achieving this apparent perfection, yet failed. Beginning with mathematics alone, he never realized his dream. However, Reason now stood as the source of meaning; the particulars finally controlled the universals. In *The Enlightenment: Studies in European History*, Roy Porter describes this titanic shift in thought for Enlightenment thinkers:

> *For a brief moment in time, the arrow pierced the barrier. Reason was now the source of meaning; the particulars finally controlled the universals.*

The *philosophes* claimed that they had dynamited obsolete religious "myths" about man... replacing them with true scientific knowledge, objectively grounded upon facts. Many historians... praise them for thus breaking with "mythopoeic" thinking, and advancing "from myth to reason."[10]

In a world following Kepler and Newton, science became the measure of all things and mathematics defined Truth. The enlightened man sought to generate meaning through experience and experiment. However, before Reason could reign supreme, the previous universals had to be destroyed. Men such as Voltaire and Rousseau rose to answer the call.

Voltaire (1694-1778)

As a central figure in the Enlightenment, the French philosopher/writer Voltaire spent his life battling the demons of Papal tyranny. His writings raged against religious intolerance though he was not intolerant of all religion, at least not initially. He held a soft spot for the peaceful English Quakers.[11] Originally Voltaire hoped to replace Christianity's dogmatism with a more tolerant "natural religion" in which a benevolent Supreme Being set Newton's mechanical universe in motion.

Many Enlightenment thinkers found religion useful. Voltaire believed a man's wife and servants should be religious—fear of eternal punishment compelled faithfulness and honesty. He quipped if God did not exist, man would have to invent Him; this kept the masses in check. However, his writings were hardly the birth of democracy. He viewed the common man as an unthinking, illiterate serf without capacity for self-government. Porter writes, "The likes of Voltaire depicted the peasantry as barely distinguishable from the beasts of the field."[12]

Similar to Plato's autonomous philosopher king, the Voltaire's elite were not subject to this Supreme Being—they were free to rule the masses. Having exalted themselves to a godlike status, they were free to establish the essence of man using Reason, even as Newton ordered the universe with mathematics. In an attempt to understand human nature the social sciences were born. Man was now defined by science.

Voltaire's view of God veered sharply to the left after a natural disaster leveled Lisbon. Following the devastating earthquake of 1755, fires and a tsunami nearly destroyed Lisbon, killing between 60,000 and 100,000 people. Ironically, Voltaire blamed the benevolent Supreme Being of his natural religion for this natural disaster. Porter describes the irony this way:

> In his last decades, Voltaire railed with restless, relentless ferocity against all religion, as though God (who after all did not exist) had done him some personal injury. His reiterated rally-call, "*Écrasez l'infâme*" [crush the infamous], was extended beyond the Pope, beyond the organized churches, to practically all manifestations of religiosity whatsoever. Voltaire ended up, perhaps, an atheist.[13]

With the help of others, Voltaire succeeded in his passionate endeavor to strip meaningful religion from France. By the end of their revolution,

Reason had expelled God from the public square. Humanism became the philosophical foundation of French society. On November 10th, 1793, as part of the <u>Festival of Reason</u>, one of the revolutionaries dressed as the Goddess of Reason and assumed the Bishop's throne in Notre Dame Cathedral. The once great Christian Cathedral was transformed into the Temple of Reason. Thomas Carlyle (a historian, scholar of the French Revolution, and mentor to Charles Dickens when Dickens wrote *A Tale of Two Cities*) reflected on these events in *The French Revolution*:

> Let the world consider it! This, O National Convention wonder of the universe, is our New Divinity, *Goddess of Reason*, worthy, and one worthy of revering. Her henceforth we adore. Nay, were it too much to ask of an august National Representation that it also went with us to the *ci-devant* Cathedral called of Notre-Dame, and executed a few strophes in worship of her?[14]

The French Revolution differed from the "Bloodless Revolution" of post-reformation England. In England, under the influence of writings such as Samuel Rutherford's *Lex Rex*, Church authority was decentralized. Power returned to the people under the "laws of nature" and the "laws of God." Those holding power were subject to both a higher law and the will of the people.

However, in France, Voltaire's humanism could not bridge the gap between the common man and the rule of law. This was an impossible task given the elite's worldview during the early Enlightenment. *Having no basis for intrinsic human worth, Voltaire viewed the commoner with disdain, incapable of democracy and self-government. The only rights the common man had were those graciously bestowed upon him by those in power. <u>This is the philosophical basis of socialism—contempt for the common man</u>.*

Government benevolence under socialism sounds so noble when first introduced. The ruling elite use sweet words of compassion to win the public's trust, even as they secure power for themselves. However, contempt for the common man lies underneath this apparent concern. We saw this with both

Barbara Wagner and Susette Kelo. In both cases the language sounded so appealing: "We will provide healthcare for the uninsured." "We will have more tax revenue to care for our citizens." Yet, in the end, the wellbeing of the citizen gave way to the welfare of the State. In the end, the elite held power.

This dichotomy between the socialism of Voltaire (which gave power to the ruling elite) and the limited government of Samuel Rutherford (*Lex Rex* returned power to the people) is clearly seen when we compare the French *Declaration of the Rights of Man* and the American *Declaration of Independence*. On August 26, 1789, only four years before the Festival of Reason (described above), the French National Assembly issued the *Declaration of the Rights of Man*. However, it could not appeal to an authority higher than its authors.

> The representatives of the French people, organized as a National Assembly, believing that the ignorance, neglect, or contempt of the rights of man are the sole cause of public calamities and of the corruption of governments, have determined to set forth in a solemn declaration the natural, unalienable, and sacred rights of man, in order that this declaration, being constantly before all the members of the Social body, shall remind them continually of their rights and duties; in order that the acts of the legislative power, as well as those of the executive power, may be compared at any moment with the objects and purposes of all political institutions and may thus be more respected, and, lastly, in order that the grievances of the citizens, based hereafter upon simple and incontestable principles, shall tend to the maintenance of the constitution and redound to the happiness of all. Therefore the National Assembly recognizes and proclaims, in the presence and under the auspices of the Supreme Being, the following rights of man and of the citizen:[15]

Having no basis for intrinsic human worth, Voltaire viewed the commoner with disdain. The only rights the common man had were those graciously bestowed upon him by those in power. This is the philosophical basis of socialism—contempt for the common man.

It is significant the last sentence asserts "the National Assembly recognizes and proclaims… the following rights of man…" Ultimately, the rights of man depended upon a governing body's appeal to Reason. This rings of Plato's philosopher king. Though "under the auspices of the Supreme Being," the intellectually elite of France were, almost entirely, either deists or atheists. If they believed in a god at all, it was a god who only set the universe in motion, leaving the affairs of man to man. Thus, appealing to an unknowable "Supreme Being" held no real meaning. Like Plato, their worldview did not contain a higher law to which the elite were bound.

Within four years of the *Declaration of the Rights of Man* came a change in power, and with a change in power came a change in ideals. Beginning in June of 1793 and lasting another thirteen months, it is estimated anywhere between 20,000 and 40,000 people were killed during the French Reign of Terror, many of them peasants. In the final month alone approximately 1,300 people were executed. It was in the middle of this Reign of Terror that Reason was enthroned at Notre Dame and God was removed from the public square.

The French *Declaration of the Rights of Man* stands in sharp contrast to the American *Declaration of Independence* written only thirteen years earlier.

> …and to assume among the powers of the earth the separate and equal station to which the laws of nature and of nature's God entitles them… We hold these truths to be self-evident, that all men are created equal, that they are endowed by their Creator with certain unalienable rights, that among these are life, liberty and the pursuit of happiness. That to secure these rights, governments are instituted among men, deriving their just powers from the consent of the governed…[16]

Our Founding Fathers' Judeo-Christian worldview understood that a knowable Creator secured man's unalienable rights. "We hold these truths to be self-evident, that all men are created equal, that they are endowed by their Creator with certain unalienable rights, that among these are life, liberty and the pursuit of happiness." The elite could neither give, nor take away, the unalienable rights of man. *(i.e.* The role of government was to protect these rights.) Because the common man had intrinsic dignity, he was capable of self-government: "That to secure these rights, governments are instituted among men, deriving their just powers from the consent of the governed..."

Man Becomes a Machine

Voltaire's Age of Reason posed another significant problem. Beginning with the assumption that only what could be proven by science and Reason was true, the *universals* were relegated to the arena of non-reason—they could not be proven scientifically. As the force of Reason strengthened and science was divorced from the Christian assumptions of Aquinas, Copernicus, Kepler, Galileo, and Newton, the *universals* of the "upper story" began to dissolve into determinism. A compassionless, purposeless, mechanical universe relentlessly pressed towards its determined end. With Newton's death, the apparent need for a personal Creator vanished

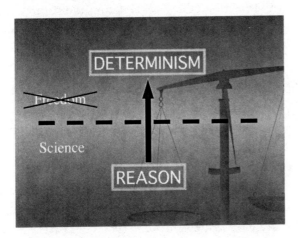

However, Newton's clocklike model of the universe was elegant, so elegant in fact that in his wake, many believed that science could explain human behavior. Man was now a system that could be understood and explained if placed under the lens of Reason—the social sciences gained new power. When the arrow broke through the barrier the formulation changed. Rather than *particulars* creating *universals, autonomous Reason* destroyed the concept of *universals,* replacing it with scientific determinism. With this transformation of worldviews, man became an insignificant cog on a remote wheel in Newton's mechanical universe. The impersonal machine of autonomous reason crushed true freedom.

The preceeding diagram clearly depicts how the French *Declaration of the Rights of Man* differs radically from the American *Declaration of Independence*. Even though *what* these documents declared was similar, *how* these two documents defended man's "unalienable" rights could not differ more. For the French, man's Reason and proclamation formed the basis for human rights, "the National Assembly recognizes and proclaims... the following rights of man..." The French used particulars in an attempt to generate universals. Their arrow pointed upward. Ultimately this meant France's rights were not unalienable, they could be revoked as easily as they had been given.

However, for America's Founding Fathers the arrow pointed downward; the universals gave meaning to the particulars. Human rights and the dignity of man were truly unalienable, bestowed upon every human by the Creator in accordance with the immutable laws of nature and nature's God. The mere fact that humans were human secured the right to "...assume among the powers of the earth the separate and equal station to which the laws of nature and of nature's God entitles them... these truths [are] self-evident, that all men are created equal, that they are endowed by their Creator with certain unalienable rights, that among these are life, liberty and the pursuit of happiness."

> The more acutely man felt the pressure of Reason forcing him into determinism, the more he felt the death of freedom.

For America's Founding Fathers the arrow pointed downward. Man's "unalienable rights" were indelibly imprinted into man himself. They could neither be given nor taken away by other men. Though written only thirteen years apart, a cavernous gulf separated the foundational philosophies of the American and the French declarations—something history never forgot.

For those following Voltaire one major difficulty remained. The more acutely man felt the pressure of Reason forcing him into determinism, the more he felt the death of freedom. *The more man believed that he was merely part of some mechanical, impersonal process the more true liberty appeared an illusion. When freedom was destroyed, pessimistic humanism was complete. Free will and autonomy were impossible. Man had become a machine.*

The consequences of autonomous Reason mandating that man is a machine are profound. Once the intrinsic dignity of man is lost, the value of life vanishes. Self worth becomes no more than a figment of imagination. Yet, man's innate desire to find meaning and true freedom is irrepressible. Before long philosophy adjusted to counter this loss of liberty because man could not live in the world he had created.

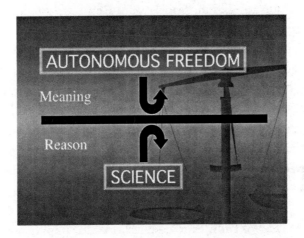

Existentialism was the eventual response. Rather than reestablishing St. Thomas's link between *universals* and *particulars* giving man intrinsic worth, the Existentialists reinforced the wall that separated the two, erased the concept of *universals*, and replaced it with *autonomous freedom*. Each individual creates the meaning of his or her own existence. Individualism reigned supreme because "Truth" was found inside each person. *Freedom became an end in itself.*

In contrast to the Enlightenment, Existentialism was not based on Reason. In fact it was the antithesis of Reason. The progression is striking. First *autonomous Reason* destroyed the universals, then man's desire for meaning destroyed Reason when applied to the upper story. The concepts of meaning and morality lost all definition as the fixed points of reference of the upper story vanished. *Autonomous freedom* reigned supreme. Where being created in God's image once gave man intrinsic value, autonomy was now the foundation of self-worth. In the lower story, science ruled unchallenged

THE BATTLE FOR AMERICA'S SOUL

over the realm of Reason becoming the definition of Truth. *Between the two stood an impenetrable wall. Any effort to link them met intense ferocity because a breach in this wall compromised autonomous freedom.*

This transformation from Enlightenment philosophy to Existentialism took nearly two centuries. Between Voltaire's concepts of pure rationalism that reduced man to a machine, and the Existentialist's concept of pure autonomy, stood five men. Each in turn revised the paradigm until freedom had no logical relationship to Reason. Jean Jacques Rousseau sought autonomy for the upper story. Immanuel Kant strengthened this autonomy by arguing that perception shaped reality. Georg Wilhelm Friedrich Hegel recast the concept of Truth altogether. Truth and falsehood were no longer mutually exclusive; they must be "synthesized" to approach a "higher truth." Søren Kierkegaard completely severed "Truth" from Reason with his leap of faith. And finally, Friedrich Nietzsche took the last step by declaring that God is dead.

The following chapter is by far the most difficult and technical of the book. However, it is necessary. It outlines the greatest shift in Western thought since the days of Plato and Aristotle. Here the reader learns how Truth died. If the reader finds this chapter too dense, the last section of the chapter, "Kierkegaard's Leap of Faith," provides a short and simplified summary.

Notes

1   Bob Hammer, *The Last Undercover: The True Story of an FBI Agent's Dangerous Dance with Evil*, Center Street Hachette Book Group, New York, New York, 2008.

2   Julie Foster, "ACLU Defends Child-Molester Group," WorldNetDaily.com, December 13, 2000.

3   Alan Sears, Craig Osten, *The ACLU vs America*, (Nashville, Tennessee: Broadman & Holman Publishers, 2005), p. 75.

4   Sarah R. Wunsch, Curley family drops case against NAMBLA, Boston Clobe Local News Update, by Jonathan Saltzman, April 23, 2008. http://www.boston.com/news/local/breaking_news/2008/04/curley_family_d.html

5   Antonio Planas, District pulls plug on speech, Reviewjournal.ocm, June 17, 2006. http://www.reviewjournal.com/lvrj_home/2006/Jun-17-Sat-2006/news/8014416.html

6   Key Cases: Brittany McComb, The Rutherford Institute, http://www.rutherford.org/keycases/mccomb.asp

7   Brittany McComb Valedictorian Speech, June 15, 2006, http://www.youtube.com/watch?v=kqzflitfHjU

8   Planas, District pulls plug on speech.

9   Nancy Pearcey, Charles Thaxton, *The Soul of Science: Christian Faith and Natural Philosophy*, (Wheaton, Illinois: Crossway Books, 1994), p. 41.

10   Roy Porter, *The Enlightenment: Studies in European History, Second Edition*, (New York: Palgrave, 2001), p. 19.

11   Ibid., p. 30.

12   Ibid., p. 25.

13   Ibid., p. 31.

14   Thomas Carlyle, *French Revolution*, http://dickens.stanford.edu/tale/issue12_gloss3.html, 2002.

15   French National Assembly, *Declaration of the Rights of Man*, 26 August, 1789.

16   United States Declaration of Independence, 4 July, 1776.

CHAPTER NINE

THE NOBLE SAVAGE

I am as free as Nature first made man…
When wild in the woods the noble savage ran.
John Dryden (1631-1700)

Rousseau and his Noble Savage

Jean Jacques Rousseau (1712-1778) knew little of his parents. His mother died shortly after his birth and his father abandoned him when he was ten. Though Swiss by birth he moved to Paris at the age of 30 where he became politically involved. In some respects this represented a kind of homecoming; his thinking fit well with the French Enlightenment. He shared their optimistic humanism and his disdain for the church was second to none. However, Rousseau rejected Enlightenment determinism becoming "the flamboyant Swiss rebel who gave birth to Romanticism. Humans [were] not part of the machine, he declared; they [were] inherently free and autonomous."[1] Autonomous freedom had found a new champion.

The early writings of Rousseau took the idea of autonomy to an extreme. In his essay *Discourse on Inequality* (1754), Rousseau cites a poem written by John Dryden a century earlier, "I am as free as Nature first made man… When wild in the woods the noble savage ran." Rousseau began with the basic assumption that primitive man was good by nature, a "noble savage," before corrupted by society and culture.

Rousseau's *Discourse on Inequality* addresses the question, "What is the origin of inequality among men?" To answer this question he believed he must first determine the nature of man. "For how shall we know the source of inequality between men, if we do not begin by knowing mankind?"[2] In many ways, this encapsulates one of the Enlightenment's primary quests—to understand human nature. How did Rousseau go about finding this answer?

As a modernist, Rousseau turns to science, the new source of Truth. He asks, "*What experiments would have to be made, to discover the natural man? And how are those experiments to be made in a state of society?*"[3] (Emphasis not added.) This perfectly exemplifies the fundamental difference between men such as Aquinas, Hooker, or Rutherford and the Enlightenment thinkers. Where the former accepted scriptural *universals*, Rousseau sets Christian thought aside. Like Descartes, he begins with the *particulars* and sets out to see what he can prove himself.

However, Rousseau found the task more difficult than it first appeared. He quickly acknowledges, "So far am I from undertaking to solve this problem, that I think I have sufficiently considered the subject, to venture to declare beforehand that our greatest philosophers would not be too good to direct such experiments, and our most powerful sovereigns to make them."[4]

This exposes the dilemma of Enlightenment thought—it could prove neither the nature of man nor his purpose. Two paragraphs later Rousseau describes this impasse:

> These investigations, which are so difficult to make, and have been hitherto so little thought of, are, nevertheless, the only means that remain of obviating a multitude of difficulties which deprive us of the knowledge of the real foundations of human society. It is this ignorance of the nature of man, which casts so much uncertainty and obscurity on the true definition of natural right: for, the idea of right... and more particularly that of natural right, are ideas manifestly relative to the nature of man.[5]

Only a few pages into the preface, Rousseau sets up an unsolvable problem. To understand human inequality we must understand human nature, the foundation of society. But human nature cannot be understood through experimentation, so we are left unable to define what is right. Thus Rousseau turns to the concept of the noble savage. He maintains that humans were good by nature before society corrupted them. Man without restraint becomes his central idea, his "Noble Savage."

Rousseau's rejection of a societal standard birthed the French Bohemian ideal. The Bohemians consisted of a loosely defined group that frequented the cafés of Paris during the early and mid-nineteenth century. They generally consisted of young artists, poets, and writers, who sought to throw off the norms of society. Because they claimed no base, they earned the name "bohemian," which meant gypsy. Their ideal? To live without restraint, *i.e.* to find *autonomous freedom.* From here thought requires only a small step to reach the Existentialism of Jaspers, Sartre, and Huxley.

One wonders how Rousseau would respond to the cannibalism of the Sawi. Free from the influences of western social pressures, the Sawi personified Rousseau's Noble Savage. But what of "fattening your enemy with friendship" before eating him? At this point even Rousseau would question his concept of complete autonomy; in reality, it did not provide a sufficient basis for culture.

The difficulty with autonomous freedom is that once limitations become necessary (one cannot eat his neighbor), who determines what those limitations should be? Without the concept of a fixed higher moral code, restraint becomes the arbitrary will of those with power.

With Rousseau's autonomous freedom, we are back to Susette Kelo's problem of a "living, breathing Constitution" under a postmodern worldview. Both lack a fixed point of reference, a higher authority to which the common man may appeal.

> *The difficulty with Rousseau's autonomous freedom is that once limitations become necessary (one cannot eat his neighbor), who determines what those limitations should be? Without the concept of a fixed higher moral code, restraint becomes the arbitrary will of those with power.*

Immanuel Kant: Truth is Redefined—The End of Enlightenment

Prior to the Enlightenment, Western culture thought in terms delineated by Aristotle and reinforced by Thomas Aquinas. Academics commonly refer to this thought form as thesis/antithesis, "A is A, it is not non-A." To the layperson this simply means that something is what it is; it is not something else. If something is true, its opposite is false. It is irrational to say both are true.

For example, if one asserts the Earth is spherical, it cannot be flat. It is nonsense to claim the Earth is a "flat sphere." Using Aristotle's thought forms, we have a clear meaning for what we observe, for Truth and non-Truth. The concepts of morality—right and wrong—fit naturally with this thought form, as do the concepts of good and evil.

Both Voltaire and Rousseau followed Aristotelian logic, yet they attacked the notion that Truth came from God. For them, Truth flowed from science. However, when humanistic thought spread northward from France to the German philosophers, Immanuel Kant and Georg Wilhelm Friedrich Hegel, Aristotelian logic itself was rejected.

Kant (1724-1804) stood one of the last of the great Enlightenment philosophers. Like Descartes, he struggled with Montaigne's question, "What do I know?" Like Voltaire, he revered Newton's clocklike universe. And like Rousseau, he felt the suffocating weight of determinism. He spent his life attempting to reconcile the world with our perception of the world. Matt McCormick of California State University sums up his work this way:

> A large part of Kant's work addresses the question "What can we know?" The answer, if it can be stated simply, is that our knowledge is constrained to mathematics and the science of the natural, empirical world. It is impossible, Kant argues, to extend knowledge to the supersensible realm of speculative metaphysics. The reason that knowledge has these constraints, Kant argues, is that the mind plays an active role in constituting the features of experience and limiting the mind's access to the empirical realm of space and time.[6]

As a scientist, Kant was enthralled by Newton's mechanical universe believing that science could understand the universe. Math and science were the languages of Truth. He wrote, it is "necessary that everything which takes place should be infallibly determined in accordance with the laws of nature."[7,8] However, Kant's "laws of nature" were far different than the "laws of nature" of Samuel Rutherford. Kant's laws were those of a mechanical universe; Rutherford's were the laws instilled by God during creation that gave meaning to man.

As a philosopher, Kant was captured by Rousseau's concept of autonomy and extended it to thought itself. Kant argued that everything we know passes through the filter of our own minds. He asserted the human mind is the originator of experience rather than the observer of it, so perception makes the reality of an object possible (in contrast to the reality of an object making perception possible). On its surface, this seems to oppose common sense. But Kant recognized our minds must decode the various sensory stimuli we constantly receive to make perception possible. Without this ability we would hear or see only "noise." Without our mind's ability to perceive, the objects themselves would be meaningless.

Notice what happened. This was the first step away from Aristotelian logic. For Kant, "reality" moved away from the object itself toward the impression it made on the mind. "Truth" depended more on the perception of the beholder than the external reality. This blurred objectivity and confused the clear delineation between the thesis and the antithesis of Aristotelian logic. If two people witnessed the same object from conflicting perspectives, there was no way to know which perception was "True." Some "Truth" was found in each perception.

Kant argued that everything we know passes through the filter of our own minds. He asserted the human mind is the originator of experience rather than the observer of it.

Problems arose when Kant attempted to mesh this view of conflicting perceptions with his strong belief that science could truly unravel the mysteries of the mechanical universe. If the mind actively generates perception, how could he guarantee the perception that scientific experimentation reflected the external reality? Kelley Ross of the Los Angeles Valley College Department of Philosophy states the difficulty this way:

But if the mind actively generates perception, this raises the question whether the result has anything to do with the world, or if so, how much... To the extent that knowledge depends on the structure of the mind and not on the world, knowledge would have no connection to the world and is not even true *representation*... Kantianism seems threatened with "psychologism," the doctrine that what we know is our own psychology, not external things.... Kant always believed that the rational structure of the mind reflected the rational structure of the world, even of things-in-themselves... But Kant had no real argument for this—the "Ideas" of reason just become "postulates" of morality—and his system leaves it as something unprovable.[9]

By initiating thought in the lower story Kant could not link knowledge, even scientific knowledge, with a certainty that it was true. This stands in contrast to the epistemology of Copernicus, Kepler, Galileo and Newton who began thought in the upper story. Like Kant, these men did not *prove* their perceptions matched reality; however, the assumption their observations indeed reflected reality logically flowed from their worldview. An intelligent God designed an ordered universe and equipped man with Reason to understand it; the two were a matched set. Man's Reason was designed to interpret the surrounding universe. This belief created the expectation the universe was "knowable" and modern science was born.

> Kant took the first step away from Aristotelian logic by blurring the meaning of "Truth." Reality moved away from the object itself toward the impression it made on the mind. In turn, "Truth" depended more on perception than the external reality.

Kant faced another dilemma with respect to moral freedom. Like Rousseau he felt the weight of determinism crushing autonomy; he understood man must be free to make moral choices if life was to have meaning. However, there was simply no way to mesh this conviction with the determinism of Newton's clocklike universe. Beginning with a mechanistic universe, Kant desperately struggled to find moral freedom for man, but he failed. In the words of Pearcey and Thaxton, for Kant,

...the lower story is what we *know*, the upper story is what we *can't help believing*.

In the end, Kant threw up his hands and simply insisted that regardless of what science says, we must act "as if" we were free. But that little phrase gives away the store: It implies that we know better, that we're tricking ourselves, and that moral freedom is little more than a useful fiction... freedom, God, and immortality "look suspiciously like pieces of wishful thinking."[10]

Kant took the first step away from Aristotelian logic by blurring the meaning of "Truth." Reality moved away from the object itself toward the impression it made on the mind. In turn, "Truth" depended more on perception than the external reality. Hegel took this transition of thought a step further—he erased the concept of Truth altogether.

The burden of autonomous Reason grew heavier, suffocating man under the weight of determinism. Not only did Kant fail to rationally create universals from the particulars, he compounded the problem. Where Rousseau erased the universals and attempted to generate his own, Kant removed the possibility of having universals by stating "Truth" is no more than a perception, not a knowable product of logic. *The hope of logically generating meaning from Reason alone faded yet further. If this dilemma could not be solved logically, then logic itself must change. Man's desire for meaning is irrepressible.*

Hegel: Truth is Dead

Kant took the first step away from Aristotelian logic by blurring the meaning of "Truth." Reality moved away from the object itself toward the impression it made on the mind. In turn, "Truth" depended more on perception than the external reality. Hegel took this transition of thought a step further—he erased the concept of Truth altogether.

The impact of Hegel's (1770-1831) writings cannot be overstated. His response to Montaigne's "What do I know?" is summarized in *The Stanford Encyclopedia of Philosophy*:

> In general this is how the *Logic* proceeds: seeking its most basic and universal determination, thought posits a category to be reflected upon [the thesis], finds then that this collapses due to a contradiction generated [antithesis], but then seeks a further category with which to make retrospective sense of that contradiction. This new category [new thesis] is more complex... But in turn the new category will generate some further contradictory negation [new antithesis] and again the demand will arise for a further concept [third thesis] which will reconcile these opposed concepts by incorporating *them* as moments.[11]

Hegel's new concept was that of "synthesis." His writing is tortuous, but the fundamental idea is that "Truth" is found by repeatedly blending the thesis and the antithesis. For Aristotle, the thesis was true and its opposite, the antithesis, was false. It was logically impossible for both to be true. For Hegel, the thesis was not entirely true and the antithesis was not entirely false. Blending these (synthesis) formed a new thesis. However, this new thesis was not entirely true and was again blended with its own antithesis yielding a third thesis. The process is then performed again, repeating itself endlessly.

Perhaps Hegel is more easily understood by applying his thinking to the case of Jeffery Curley and the ACLU mentioned at the beginning of chapter eight. In the thought form of thesis/antithesis the argument is framed:

Thesis #1: Advocating the homosexual rape of young boys is wrong. Antithesis #1: The right to free speech is the supreme good to be protected above all else. Aristotelian logic maintains that if the thesis is true the antithesis is false. If advocating the rape of young boys is wrong (this represents an absolute) then there must be limits of free speech (the antithesis is false). Hegel on the other hand rejects this absolutist way of thinking. He maintains the thesis is not completely true and the antithesis is not completely false; Truth is approached by blending the two. Hegel might suggest this:

Thesis #2: Forcing a boy to have sex with a man is always harmful to the boy's future, but there is a right of free speech to advocate this perspective, however misguided. This statement in turn has its own antithesis. Antithesis #2: It is not always harmful for men to have sex with boys. Blending this with Thesis #2 results in Thesis #3.

Thesis #3: Sexual relationships between young boys and men are often harmful to a boys psychological health, but there may be times a boy may find comfort in this relationship and given his right to self determination, may choose this behavior. To advocate such beneficial relationships is not only not wrong, but to be commended.

Notice what happened. Hegel's concept of synthesis turned the original thesis, "Advocating the homosexual rape of young boys is wrong," on its head. By the time we reach Thesis #3 we actually commend the very thing we began saying was categorically wrong. Hegel's thought form of "synthesis" revolutionized logic and shook the world. Truth died for all who followed in Hegel's footsteps.[12]

Using Hegel's reasoning we actually end by commending the very thing we began saying was categorically wrong. This is why Truth died for all who followed in Hegel's footsteps.

Finding Truth for any of life's ultimate questions suddenly became logically impossible for the intellectually astute. Those who claimed to know "moral certainty" bore the mark of ultimate naiveté. It was not long until the impact of Hegel's philosophy was fully felt with the dawning of existentialism.

Kierkegaard's Leap of Faith

So we find a progression of Enlightened thought. Voltaire sought unity of the upper and lower story through pure Reason but ended only having destroyed the previous universals. Rousseau rebutted the dilemma of Voltaire's mechanical universe by placing autonomous freedom in the upper story. Kant wanted to believe there was a relationship between reality and knowledge, but he further weakened the logical relationship between the upper and lower stories by asserting perceptions shaped reality. "Truth" was now in the mind of the beholder. Finally, Hegel could not rationally unite the universals and the particulars, so he recast Reason altogether. "Truth" no longer rationally existed; it could only be approached.

Each of these men had one thing in common: they struggled to rationally unite the upper and lower stories. All searched for a rational way to find the universals of life. Man's thirst for meaning was unquenchable; Hegel even altered logic itself to find an answer for this unsolved mystery. But the solution that escaped these great men awaited the Danish philosopher and theologian Søren Kierkegaard (1813-1855). Where Voltaire, Rousseau, Kant, and Hegel all failed, Kierkegaard succeeded—but only by removing the question.

With Kierkegaard came another tremendous shift in thought. Previously, philosophers focused on Montaigne's question, "What do I know?" They sought to produce metaphysical systems that explained reality and knowledge. But Kierkegaard believed philosophy should focus on the human experience, man's existence. In doing so he became the "Father of Existentialism."

In many ways, Kierkegaard paralleled Descartes, only removed by 200 years. Both were deeply religious. Both used powerful intellects to reconcile faith with the world they knew. Both marked the end of an age and set in motion an unintended revolution of thought for the age to come.

> *What man cannot do, Kierkegaard believed, was to come to God by virtue of Reason. To have faith was to abandon Reason. To have faith was to believe in the absurd.*

When Descartes reversed the once downward pointing arrow, he opened the door for the Enlightenment. For the two centuries following Descartes thinkers attempted to tie the upper story to the lower story by generating universals based on Reason. Kierkegaard, however, ushered in Existentialism when he made the line between the upper and lower stories impenetrable. For the two centuries following Kierkegaard the universals were relegated to the arena of non-Reason.

The intensely introspective Kierkegaard blended theology, psychology, and philosophy in his search for meaning and significance. He moved past Enlightenment thought in that he no longer coveted autonomy. He yearned once again to find the meaning of existence. In response to Hegel's impersonal philosophy, Kierkegaard sought to regain individuality by emphasizing the importance of personal significance.

Kierkegaard maintained that the pleasures of life (esthetics) are short-lived leading to despair. If man then turned to social ethics he found a sense of permanence but, as this was only partial, man again confronted despair. Kierkegaard believed that only when man moved to the level of religion did he find permanence and meaning. By religion, Kierkegaard does not mean the mere recitation of church dogma but a personal passion for God. For Kierkegaard faith is the most important task for humans to achieve. However, at this level he believed that Reason fell short.

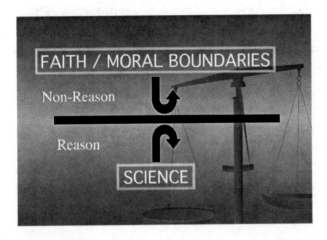

Running through Kierkegaard's writings are the paradoxes of Christianity. The transcendent, infinite, eternal God was born as a finite, temporal, son of a carpenter. The same God who asked Abraham to kill his own son Isaac later commanded Israel to not murder. In dealing with the God of Christianity, Kierkegaard found paradoxes that lay beyond Reason. Here man faced a choice: to be intellectually offended and reject the concept of God or to set Reason aside and approach God with an irrational faith. What man cannot do, Kierkegaard believed, was to come to God by virtue of Reason. *To have faith was to abandon Reason. To have faith was to believe in the absurd. With Kierkegaard, we return to Siger of Brabant and the double mined man.*

Notice what happened with Kierkegaard's formulation. The upper story containing the universals, the meaning of life, and the concept of moral restraint was divorced from Reason. It moved into the realm of non-Reason where it could only be accessed through faith. However, faith was no longer Reasonable; faith was now irrational. Though Kierkegaard by no means intended to destroy religion, he could not have found better nails with which to seal Christianity's coffin. Once declared irrational, Judeo-Christian was soon marginalized from society. Like Descartes, Kierkegaard destroyed the very thing he loved.

Once the intellectually elite banished Judeo-Christian thought to the realm of non-Reason, to use the concept of moral boundaries to limit the *autonomous freedom* not only incited contempt but rage. No one displayed this more than a brilliant, late nineteenth century philosopher. His writings exposed the fiery passion behind the growing conflict. He vividly articulated one side of a battle that had been brewing for over a century. So strong was the influence of this passionate German that Martin Heidegger once said that since his time, all thinking has gone on in his shadow.

Who was this man? None other than Friedrich Nietzsche.

Notes

1   Pearcey, Thaxton, p. 104

2   Jean Jacques Rousseau, *Discourse on Inequality*, Preface, online text, www. constitution.org/jjr/ineq.htm

3   Ibid.

4   Ibid.

5   Ibid.

6   Matt McCormick, *Immanuel Kant (1724-1804) Metaphysics*, The Internet Encyclopedia of Philosophy, www.iep.utm.edu/k/kantmeta.htm, November, 2005.

7   Immanuel Kant, Groundwork of the Metaphysics of Morals, (New York: Harper & Row, 1964), pp. 116, 123.

8   Pearcey, Thaxton, p. 104.

9   Kelly Ross, *Immanuel Kant*, www.friesian.com/kant.htm

10   Pearcey, Thaxton, pp. 105, 106.

11   Redding, Paul, "Georg Wilhelm Friedrich Hegel", *The Stanford Encyclopedia of Philosophy (Summer 2002 Edition)*, Edward N. Zalta (ed.), URL = <http://plato. stanford.edu/archives/sum2002/entries/hegel/>

12   Schaeffer, *Volume 5: How Should We then Live?*, pp. 178-179.

CHAPTER TEN

NIETZSCHE'S LION UNLEASHED

The will to power can express itself only against resistances;
it seeks that which resists it.

Friedrich Nietzsche (1844-1900)

The *Day After Tomorrow* is a science fiction film depicting a cataclysmic climate shift. Global warming melts the polar ice cap disrupting the North Atlantic current. As a result, super-cooled air from the upper troposphere pouring into the atmosphere plunges the Earth headlong into another ice age. Trapped in a New York City library, survivors burn books to stave off the plummeting temperatures, hoping against all odds that help arrives in time. Though compromised by its political agenda, the film's focus on the rescue of two specific books is noteworthy.

The first volume salvaged contains the works of Nietzsche. Picking up the book the actor earnestly states, "Friedrich Nietzsche. We cannot burn Friedrich Nietzsche. He was the most important thinker of the nineteenth century."

Several hours later, a romantic fire flickers in the background. The same actor sits in a chair clutching another book. Intrigued, a woman asks, "What have you got there?"

Staring at his treasured volume he replies, "A Gutenberg Bible. It was in the rare books room."

Without sarcasm she inquires, "You think God is going to save you?"

"No." Lifting his eyes, his tone is measured and confident. "I don't believe in God."

"You're holding on to that Bible pretty tight?" She remains unconvinced.

"I'm protecting it," the man states with intellectual certainty. He then pauses for a moment to reflect on the gravity of the situation. With carefully chosen words the man continues, "This Bible is the first book ever printed. It represents the dawn of the Age of Reason. As far as I am concerned, the written word is mankind's greatest achievement. You can laugh. But if western civilization is finished, I'm going to save at least one little piece of it."

Why preserve these two particular volumes as modern civilization is coming to an end? Why not the *Declaration of Independence* or the *United States Constitution*? The answer? Whether or not the scriptwriters realized it, these two writings portray the bookends of all human thought. Having examined the tremendous philosophical and political influence of the Gutenberg Bible in chapter four, we must now turn to the works of Nietzsche.

> Where Enlightenment thinkers placed religion in the category of non-Reason Nietzsche erased the concept of God altogether.

Beyond Good and Evil

Psychiatrist and Holocaust survivor Victor Frankl once said, "He who has a *why* to live can bear almost any *how*." [1,2] In his book *Man's Search for Meaning*, one ironically finds that Frankl was quoting a man who was profoundly anti-Semitic, a man whose philosophy fueled the prison camp in which he sat. Who was this man? None other than Friedrich Nietzsche.

Son of a Lutheran clergyman, Nietzsche (1844-1900) was born near Leipzig. He was an exceptionally bright man, becoming the chair of classical philology at Basel University at age 23. He remained there until poor health compelled him to retire twelve years later. Nietzsche wrote for another eleven years before what was likely neurosyphilis forced him to enter an insane asylum at age 46. There he suffered for another ten tormented years, dying as a new century began.

Nietzsche's place in the flow of history helps the reader understand the significance of what he wrote. A century earlier, Rousseau (1712-1778) threw off societal restraint with his "Noble Savage." Fifty years earlier, Kierkegaard (1813-1855) drew an impenetrable line separating the *universals* from the *particulars* with his "leap of faith." By equating faith with non-Reason, Kierkegaard positioned morality and religion to draw the intellectual's scorn—something not long in coming. Nietzsche expressed it this way, "The entire realm of morality and religion falls under this concept of imaginary causes."[3]

Where Enlightenment thinkers placed religion in the category of non-Reason Nietzsche erased the concept of God altogether. The result? The academically elite despised those who believed in a moral code defined by God. As far as modern thinkers were concerned, only fools believed in moral certainty. The concepts of good and evil were mere illusions. Here we begin to see pressure building that would nearly drive conservative thought out of academics altogether. In *Twilight of the Idols* Nietzsche makes this position clear:

> One knows my demand of philosophers that they place themselves *beyond* good and evil—that they have the illusion of moral judgement *beneath* them. This demand follows from an insight first formulated by me: *that there are no moral facts whatever*. Moral judgement has this in common with religious judgement that it believes in realities which do not exist. Morality is only an interpretation of certain phenomena, more precisely a *mis*interpretation. Moral judgement belongs, as does religious judgement, to a level of ignorance at which even the concept of the real, the distinction between the real and the imaginary, is lacking: so that at such a level 'truth' denotes nothing but things which we today call 'imaginings'. To this extent moral judgement is never to be taken literally: as such it never contains anything but nonsense.[4]

Between Kierkegaard and Nietzsche lay Charles Darwin (1809-1882). Published in 1859, *The Origin of Species* provided the final piece needed to complete the puzzle of humanism—man could now rid himself of God entirely and remain intellectually honest. For the first time, Darwinian evolution laid out a plausible scientific theory of man's existence without the direct intervention of a Supreme Being. Enlightenment philosophy was based on this assumption but lacked scientific evidence. As anthropologist Richard Dawkins remarked, Darwin finally "made it possible to be an intellectually fulfilled atheist."[5] Following in Darwin's footsteps, Nietzsche no longer needed Kierkegaard's "leap of faith." He dispensed with God altogether.

"God is Dead," is perhaps the most famous of Nietzsche's quotations. This concept is developed in one of his earliest works, *The Gay Science* (1882).

> God is dead: but as the human race is constituted, there will perhaps be caves for millenniums yet, in which people will show his shadow. And we—we have still to overcome his shadow![6]

Near the middle of the book Nietzsche expands on this discussion:

> Where is God gone? ...I mean to tell you! We have killed him, you and I! We are all his murderers! ...Does not empty space breathe upon us? Has it not become colder? Does not night come on continually, darker and darker? Shall we not have to light lanterns in the morning? Do we not hear the noise of the grave-diggers who are burying God? Do we not smell the divine putrefaction?—for even Gods putrefy! God is dead! God remains dead! And we have killed him! ...Is not the magnitude of this deed too great for us? Shall we not ourselves have to become Gods, merely to seem worthy of it? There never was a greater event—and on account of it, all who are born after us belong to a higher history than any history hitherto!
>
> ...What are these churches now, if they are not the tombs and monuments of God?[7]

Nietzsche's Lion Destroys the Moral Code

In *Thus Spoke Zarathustra* (1883), Nietzsche proposed that the task of humanity is to elevate one's self and to create new values. Near the beginning of this book he uses an allegory to explain the development of man's spirit. This process requires three stages: 1) A Camel, 2) A Lion, and 3) A child.

—First the spirit of mankind becomes a camel, a beast of burden. The camel carries the afflictions of humanity (which Nietzsche views as submission to Judeo-Christian morality) into a desert. However, the camel cannot destroy what so encumbers mankind. The camel must transform itself into a lion, capable of killing whatever stands in the way of freedom.

—The lion battles a great dragon covered with scales of golden "Thou Shalts," referencing the Old Testament's Ten Commandments. By killing the dragon, the lion destroys the old moral code. Yet, the lion itself cannot actually create new values; rather, it provides the opportunity for this to be done. The lion must transform itself into a child.

—Not having known the restraints of the previous "Thou Shalts," the child is free to create new values of his own. Nietzsche viewed this as the great liberation of mankind, the new door of human emancipation—his sea without a shore.[8] Not one for humility, Nietzsche claimed *Thus Spoke Zarathustra* as the greatest book the world had ever seen. Indeed, his work marked the end of an age.

This allegory represents some of Nietzsche's best writing. Though not intended to do so, it concisely depicts the process that took place between 1500 and 1850. Then, in an almost prophetic fashion, the allegory also portrays what was to happen between 1898 and 1973 with the rise of Existentialism. Like the camel, the Renaissance isolated Christianity from its foundations as men like da Vinci and Descartes began thought with the *particulars* rather than the *universals*. Taking the role of the lion, Enlightenment thinkers such as Voltaire and Rousseau (ending with Nietzsche himself) destroyed the foundations of Christianity by separating faith and Reason, drawing an impenetrable line between the upper and lower stories, and then removing God. Finally the child arrived. Existentialist thinkers such as Sartre, Jaspers, and Huxley built a new upper story where *autonomous freedom* roamed without restraint. With the dragon slain, Existential thinkers melted the golden "Thou Shalts" and forged them into the imaginings of man.

Nietzsche looks back at what the death of God means:

> Indeed, we philosophers and "free spirits" feel, when we hear the news that the "old god is dead," as if a new dawn shone on us; our heart overflows with gratitude, amazement, premonitions, expectation. At long last the horizon appears free to us again, even if it should not be bright; at long last our ships may venture out again, venture out to face any danger; all the daring of the lover of knowledge is permitted again; the sea, *our* sea, lies open again; perhaps there has never yet been such an "open sea."[9]

Nietzsche's Open Sea of Autonomous Freedom

With all boundaries removed Nietzsche gazed upon the unbroken horizon with breathless delight. No shores loomed to confine his course; no island arose to limit where he sailed! Driven by the winds of passion and powered by the engine of Darwinian science, he relished the *autonomous freedom* found on his open sea. Without a God, he was free to chase his imaginings wherever they led. No one would deny him this freedom again, of that he was certain.

At last mankind is free! Moral restraint has been destroyed! While Nietzsche's defiance was new, he actually marked the end of a long transition. The process of displacing God from the upper story, erasing the *universals*, and erecting an impenetrable wall between faith and Reason had been in transition for more than two centuries. Nietzsche was the capstone, the voice proclaiming final victory. Without the influence of God, religion, and faith, Reason was now without imposition or restraint and science was free to rule in the realm of Reason. By pronouncing God dead, Nietzsche opened the door to recreate morality, the greatest task man could undertake.

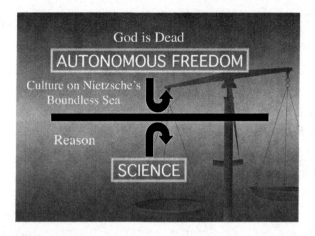

The social impact of moving from thinkers such as Aquinas or Rutherford (men who began with the assumption of a real God that was involved in human affairs) to Kierkegaard, and finally to Nietzsche, was profound. To understand this transition a classroom analogy is helpful. If a teacher actively sets limits in a classroom, behavior is restrained (i.e. Rutherford's "laws of nature" and "laws of God"). If the teacher remains in the room, but the children are told there will be no discipline, the children will do things they previously would not (i.e. Kierkegaard's impenetrable wall). However, even if the teacher only watches the children, their behavior will be partially restrained as they retain the memory of discipline; the children are only *partially autonomous*. Now remove the teacher altogether and leave the children completely unsupervised (i.e. Nietzsche, God is dead). This is *autonomous freedom*.

> Nietzsche charges that Christianity fraudulently maintains there is an "equality of souls before God." This profound concept pierces heart of American political philosophy.

For Nietzsche, the influence of the Judeo-Christian God represented mankind's greatest travesty, the blemish on freedom's cloudless horizon. He viewed religion as a corrupting illusion intended to render the powerful impotent and held the Judeo-Christian moral code with more disdain than did even Voltaire or Rousseau. He took it upon himself to set mankind free from the vestiges of religious bondage and moral restraint.

Nietzsche Rages Against Moral Restraint to Find Freedom: But Freedom for Whom?

Out of Nietzsche's struggle for moral autonomy arose a loathing of Judaism and Christianity. Jews and Christians surrendered final moral authority to God in a fashion similar to Hippocrates. Nietzsche seized moral authority for those in power following in the footsteps of Plato. (Both Nietzsche and Plato believed the value of human life was determined by those in power, not unlike the elite during the French Revolution.)

In his writings, Nietzsche's contempt for women is shocking. He quipped, "When a woman has scholarly inclinations, there is usually something wrong with her sexuality,"[10] and "Stupidity in the kitchen; woman as cook."[11] However, he reserved his deepest vitriol for Jews and Christians, particularly Christians. Nietzsche's scorn flares in the last section of one of the last books he wrote, *The AntiChrist*:

> With this I come to a conclusion and pronounce my judgment. I *condemn* Christianity; I bring against the Christian church the most terrible of all the accusations that an accuser has ever had in his mouth. It is, to me, the greatest of all imaginable corruptions; it seeks to work the ultimate corruption, the worst possible corruption. The Christian church has left nothing untouched by its depravity; it has turned every value into worthlessness, and every truth into a lie, and every integrity into baseness of soul. Let any one dare to speak to me of its "humanitarian" blessings! Its deepest necessities range it against any effort to abolish distress; it lives by distress; it *creates* distress to make *itself* immortal.... For example, the worm of sin: it was the church that first enriched mankind with this misery!—**The "equality of souls before God"—this fraud, this *pretext* for the *rancors* of all the base-minded—this explosive concept, ending in revolution, the modern idea, and the notion of overthrowing the whole social order—this is *Christian* dynamite...**

This eternal accusation against Christianity I shall write upon all walls, wherever walls are to be found—I have letters that even the blind will be able to see.... I call Christianity the one great curse, the one great intrinsic depravity, the one great instinct of revenge, for which no means are venomous enough, or secret, subterranean and *small* enough,—I call it the one immortal blemish upon the human race...[12] (emphasis in bold added.)

Nietzsche held Judaism and Christianity in such contempt for reasons different than Voltaire and Rousseau. Where the latter were driven by the abuses of the church, Nietzsche fought for *autonomous freedom*. He contended, "The concept 'God' has hitherto been the greatest *objection* to existence.... We deny God; in denying God, we deny accountability: only by doing *that* do we redeem the world."[13] Nietzsche struggled to "redeem the world" by removing all restraint. However, redeem the world for whom?

Nietzsche charges that Christianity fraudulently maintains there is an "equality of souls before God" (bold quotation above). This profound concept pierces heart of the philosophical foundations for political systems and culture. As noted in previous chapters, the bedrock of the *Declaration of Independence* is the equality of man before God... "which the laws of nature and of nature's God entitles them... We hold these truths to be self-evident, that all men are created equal, that they are endowed by their Creator with certain unalienable rights, that among these are life, liberty and the pursuit of happiness." Accepting the "laws of nature a and laws of God" as reality provides the philosophical foundation for the concept that no human, no matter what position of political power he or she holds, has the ability to either give or take away these unalienable rights. To destroy God is to destroy this foundatin.

> Where the Declaration of Independence maintains all men are created equal, Nietzsche asserts they are not. Nietzsche's position? "Independence is for the very few; it is a privilege of the strong."

Where the *Declaration of Independence* maintains all men are created equal, Nietzsche asserts they are not. In *Beyond Good and Evil*, Nietzsche *addresses this specifically, "Independence is for the very few; it is a privilege of the strong."*[14]

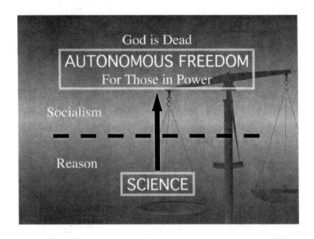

Notice what has happened. Our Founding Fathers began with the premise of man's innate equality before God. The result? They created world's longest ongoing constitutional republic based on the rule of law. Nietzsche declared God dead rejecting the reality of moral truth. The result? His autonomous freedom did not extend to those in need; they received little more than contempt. We saw this previously in the ideas of Voltaire. As Porter noted, "The likes of Voltaire depicted the peasantry as barely distinguishable from the beasts of the field."[15] Without God, those in power turned to Science as their Reason for rule.

Judeo-Christian thought placed eternal significance on the common man and actions of this life, urging love and compassion for the poor and needy. Nietzsche despised the poor and needy. He believed the weak manipulated morality to subdue the strong through guilt. Contrary to traditional norms of western civilization, Nietzsche understood "good" to be whatever was strong, powerful, and self-sufficient. He viewed traits such as compassion, love, pity, and altruism as weaknesses to be despised above all else and ultimately "evil." In *Twilight of the Idols*, Nietzsche states:

> What is good?—All that heightens the feeling of power, the will to power, power itself in man.

What is bad?—All that proceeds from weakness.

What is happiness?—the feeling that power increases…

The weak and ill-constituted shall perish: first principle of our philanthropy. And one shall help them to do so.

What is more harmful than any vice?—Active sympathy for the ill-constituted and weak—Christianity…[16]

Pronouncing God dead created a tremendous philosophical vacuum. The universals of humanity were suddenly up for grabs. There would be law—of that there was no doubt. The question was, "Whose law would it be?" Nietzsche believed that whoever created the new values for society required abundant health and strength. He used the term *übermensch* (often translated "overman") to describe an individual who overcomes traditional values and rises above humanity to establish a new morality—the law of the elite. This is the philosophical base of modern day socialism. Freed from the concept of a higher moral code, the elite legislate values for the rest of society. What is legal now defines what is "right" and those in power now determine the value of the weak and infirm. Law determines morality rather than morality determining law. This is Nietzsche's "will to power." In *Beyond Good and Evil* he states:

> Genuine philosophers, however, are commanders and legislators: they say, "*thus* it *shall* be!" They first determine the Whither and For What of man… With a creative hand they reach for the future, and all that is and has been becomes a means for them, an instrument, a hammer. Their "knowing" is *creating*, their creating is a legislation, their will to truth is—*will to power*.[17]

To realize his will to power and his "first principle of philanthropy" (letting the weak and ill-constituted perish), Nietzsche specifically addressed the role of the physician. History had come full circle. By recreating the world of ancient Greece Nietzsche resurrected Plato's philosopher king.

Notes

1   Viktor Frankl, *Man's Search for Meaning*, (New York: Simon and Schuster, Third Edition, 1984), p. 9.

2   Friedrich Nietzsche, *Twilight of the Idols / The AntiChrist*, translated by R. J. Hollingdale (New York & Toronto: Penguin Books, 1990), p. 33.

3   Ibid., p. 63.

4   Ibid., p. 66.

5   Richard Dawkins, *The Blind Watchmaker*, (New York: W.W.Norton & Company, 1996), p. 6.

6   Friedrich Nietzsche, *The Gay Science*, section 108.

7   Ibid., section 125.

8   Friedrich Nietzsche, *Thus Spoke Zarathustra*, translated by Walter Kaufmann, (New York & London: Penguin Books, 1966), pp. 25-27.

9   Nietzsche, *The Gay Science*, section 343.

10   Friedrich Nietzsche, *Beyond Good & Evil*, translated by Walter Kaufmann, (New York: Vintage Books, 1966), p. 89.

11   Ibid., p. 164.

12   Friedrich Nietzsche, *The Anti-Christ*, translated by H. L. Mencken, (Tucson, AZ: See Sharp Press, 1999), pp. 90-91.

13   Friedrich Nietzsche, *Twilight of the Idols*, p. 65.

14   Friedrich Nietzsche, *Beyond Good & Evil*, p. 41.

15   Ibid., p. 25.

16   Ibid., pp. 127-128.

17   Friedrich Nietzsche, *Beyond Good & Evil*, p. 136.

CHAPTER ELEVEN

NIETZSCHE'S PHYSICIAN: RETURNING TO ANCIENT GREECE WITH CONTEMPT

The invalid is a parasite on society.
In a certain state it is indecent to go on living.
To vegetate on in a cowardly dependence on physicians and medicaments
after the meaning of life, the right to life, has been lost
ought to entail the profound contempt of society.
Physicians, in their turn, ought to be the
communicators of this contempt.

Friedrich Nietzsche (1844-1900)

Nietzsche and Plato held similar underlying worldviews. Nietzsche gave power to his overman, Plato to his philosopher king. Because both removed power from the common man and gave it to the elite, it comes as no surprise they reached similar conclusions. In reading Twilight of the Idols we find that Nietzsche specifically addressed the physician's role in society. Two sections from this book reveal unmistakable parallels with the thinking of Plato. Nietzsche sates:

Section 33: The natural value of egoism.
Every individual may be regarded as representing the

ascending or descending line of life. When one has decided
which, one has thereby established a canon for the value of
his egoism. If he represents the ascending line his value is
in fact extraordinary—and for the sake of the life-collective,
which with him takes a step *forward*, the care expended on
his preservation, on the creation of optimum conditions for
him, may even be extreme... If he represents the descending
development, decay, chronic degeneration, sickening...
then he can be accorded little value, and elementary fairness
demands that he *takes away* as little as possible from the well-
constituted. He is not better than a parasite on them...[1]

Section 36: A moral code for physicians.
The invalid is a parasite on society. In a certain state it
is indecent to go on living. To vegetate on in a cowardly
dependence on physicians and medicaments after the
meaning of life, the *right* to life, has been lost ought to
entail the profound contempt of society. Physicians, in their
turn, ought to be the communicators of this contempt—
not prescriptions, but every day a fresh dose of *disgust* with
their patients... To create a new responsibility, that of the
physician, in all cases in which the highest interest of life,
of *ascending* life, demands the most ruthless suppression
and sequestration of degenerating life—for example in
determining the right to reproduce, the right to be born, the
right to live...[2]

This clearly rings of Plato, and indeed Nietzsche had read his works.[3] It
is worth quoting Plato again for comparison.

...but bodies which disease had penetrated through and
through [the physician] would not have attempted to cure...
he did not want to lengthen out good-for-nothing lives, or
to have weak fathers begetting weaker sons;—if a man was

not able to live in the ordinary way [the physician] had no business to cure him; for such a cure would have been of no use either to himself, or to the State...[4]

"So at the same time as legislating for this type of legal practice in our community, you'll also legislate for the kind of medical practice we described. These two practices will treat the bodies and minds of those of your citizens who are naturally well endowed in these respects; as for the rest, those with a poor physical constitution will be allowed to die, and those with irredeemably rotten minds will be put to death. Right?"

"Yes, we've shown that this is the best course," he said, "for those at the receiving end of the treatment as well as for the community."[5]

As shocking as these positions are we must ask, "Are they so different from the Oregon Health Plan's treatment of Barbara Wagner? Are they so different from the thinking of Peter Singer, one of the most prominent bioethicists in America?" Stripping God from culture strips man of meaning. Without a "higher law" those in power determine the "right." As we will see later, America is witnessing a steady and concerted effort to remove God from the public square. If this effort is successful, why should we expect American medicine to end differently than what Plato, Nietzsche, and Singer envision? Americans must recognize those who most strongly strive to remove God from culture are largely the same people who clamber for "universal healthcare." Driven by a common underlying worldview, ideas tend to move together and history shows us where this road may end.

Cheers and accolades greet the thought of government ensuring healthcare for every American. However, we must ask, "Who should control the personal

Cheers and accolades greet the thought of government ensuring healthcare for every American. However, we must ask, "Who should control the personal and complex process of medical decision-making? The patient and the patient's family together with his or her physician? Or the State?"

and complex process of medical decision-making? The patient and the patient's family together with his or her physician? Or the State?" Americans must be aware, *whoever pays holds the power to choose and the government cannot afford to pay for everything for everyone.* Barbara Wagner learned this only too well. Remember, two worldviews struggle for control of America—one empowers and protects the individual; one surrenders power to the State. Which path will we choose? Will we follow Plato or Hippocrates?

The core medical ethics of Plato and Nietzsche were nearly identical. Why? These views are the logical conclusions to their similar underlying worldviews. Neither believed in the sanctity of human life nor in the supreme commitment of the physician to the patient. Both used the physician as a tool of the state. Neither saw value in treating the infirm and believed it was better to kill the weak or let them die. Plato believed this was essential to create the ideal state; Nietzsche believed this was essential to create the ideal race. These moral codes for physicians were nearly identical because both Nietzsche and Plato worked for a worldview with one essential commonality: *the worldviews of both men lacked a fixed point by which all things could be judged. They lacked a moral code to which the ruling elite must submit.*

> Americans must be aware, whoever pays holds the power to choose and the government cannot afford to pay for everything for everyone.

What Thomas Aquinas had foreseen in his debate with Siger of Brabant had finally come true. The use of Aristotle's Reason that Aquinas had fought so hard to integrate into Christian thought had destroyed the very thing he loved. In the end, this stripped man of meaning and opened the door of unfettered freedom to the elite. The few finally attained *autonomous power* and the common man was left without recourse.

Why bother with metaphysics and philosophy? Because the ideas of men shape their actions. Science and philosophy were about to merge to form social policy.

Medicine in Nazi Germany

In less than 50 years following his death, Nietzsche's philosophy had seized the German culture, culminating with Nazi tyranny. Hitler filled the role of Nietzsche's allegorical child. Using the medical community as a tool to eliminate those perceived as weak, Hitler sought to develop a pure and powerful race through genetic purification. In fact, Hitler embodied Nietzsche's "will to power." Drawing on the work of Charles Darwin (1809-1882), this "will to power" fueled much of what transpired in Germany during those dark years. However, the idea of Aryan supremacy, Jewish culpability, and loss of the sanctity of life did not begin with Hitler; it existed in German culture prior to Hitler's rise to power.

The medical atrocities of the German concentration camps had roots reaching back to the early 1900's. In his book *Murderous Science*, Benno Müller-Hill recounts events in German medicine, politics, and law. Muller-Hill begins his chronicle with the rediscovery of Darwin's contemporary, Gregor Mendel (1822-1884), the "Father of Genetics," in 1900. The explosive combination of Mendel's brilliant work in genetics, Darwin's captivating theory of the survival of the fittest, the growing philosophical commitment to scientific autonomy, and Nietzsche's vitriolic contempt for the weak, all led to one of the greatest horrors of human history.

Muller-Hill begins his book with a timeline of events between 1900 and May 8, 1945, World War II:

1900—The work of Mendel is rediscovered. Those who regard traits such as intelligence are inherited believe their hypothesis is scientifically proved by Mendelian genetics. For them the whole of human history becomes part of Darwinian evolution. They see it as their duty to demand the prevention of procreation by "other inferior races."

1918—Half of the patients in German mental hospitals die from hunger and infectious disease.

1920—The jurist Professor Binding and psychiatrist Professor Hoche published *The Sanctioning of the Destruction of Lives Unworthy to be Lived*.

1924—Hitler reads *The Principles of Human Heredity and Race-Hygiene* eventually using some of these radical ideas in *Mein Kampf*.

1931—SS troops (the *Schutzstaffel*, literally the "defense squadron," the elite Nazi secret police led by Heinrich Himmler) must obtain permission from the newly established Race Bureau in order to marry. Permission is granted based upon race and hereditary health.

1933—Hitler becomes Chancellor of the Third Reich.

1933—The "Law for the Prevention of Progeny with Hereditary Defects" is proclaimed allowing the compulsory sterilization of individuals with mental defects, schizophrenia, manic-depression, epilepsy, and severe alcoholism.

1934—At the Expert Advisory Council for Population and Race Policy, Professor Lenz states, "As things are now, it is only a minority of our fellow citizens who are so endowed that their unrestricted procreation is good for the race."

1937—German children of color are marked for compulsory sterilization.

1939—Hitler invades Poland beginning World War II and introduces euthanasia at the hands of specially designated physicians. By September, 1941, more than 70,000 psychiatric patients have been killed using carbon monoxide.

1941—Germany declares war on the United States.

1943—Himmler decrees that only physicians trained in anthropology are to select patients for extermination and supervise their killing.

1945—World War II ends leaving six million Jews dead.[6]

Not only was the physician of Plato's ideal state reincarnated, he took on a life of his own. No longer bound to Plato's goal of a moral and virtuous life, the new physician practiced his art free from moral constraint—Nietzsche's allegorical child now ruled. The story of medical atrocities continued into the German concentration camps. Recall the Dachau Hypothermia Experiments lowered men into ice water to see how long it would take them to freeze to death. Before some died they were "rewarmed," using various methods including vats of boiling water to determine the optimum method for treating hypothermic pilots.

As another example, after his capture, Claude J. Letulle testified: "I was captured by the German army six weeks after they invaded France. Like other POWs, I was put to forced work for the Reich. As punishment for threatening to kill a guard, I was made to work in a hospital where Nazi doctors performed 'medical experiments.' I was present when they castrated men, and when they crushed prisoners' fingers in a press to 'study' broken bones. Many died during the procedures. One woman's eyelids were sewn open to force her to watch in a mirror as both her breasts were removed."[7]

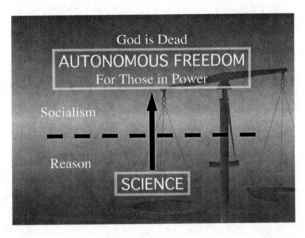

God was dead, killed by Nietzsche's lion. Reason and scientific objectivity reigned supreme, praising themselves for not succumbing to the irrationality of value judgments. But the price of pure objectivity was high; all possible outcomes must be feasible—even the experiments, the ovens, and the mass graves. No external limits existed to warn of oncoming disaster. If economics demanded the sacrifice of tens of thousands of mentally ill, Reason demanded it must be so. If the "good of a nation" required genocide, who could protest? Scientific objectivity in a world without boundaries ended in barbarism. Divorced from the universals, science now lay cold and emotionless, stripping the common man of meaning. Man finally achieved *autonomous freedom*, but was he free? Or had the machine of modern science consumed him?

Nietzsche's ideas and the prevailing German thought of the 1920s, 30s and 40s had many similarities. Both forsook a higher moral code. Both renounced the sanctity of life. Both held Jews liable for the problems of the day. Both believed in the extermination of the weak and deformed. Both believed in the rise of the German *übermensch*. Nietzsche wrote of these things; Hitler's Germany carried them out. More important than any individual similarity between Plato, Nietzsche, and Hitler, we must recognize the common threads woven throughout their worldviews.

When man has no *universals* and begins with only the *particulars*, all moral boundaries are removed. Fyodor Dostoevsky succinctly stated the result, "Without God, all things are lawful."[8] Where it is acknowledged that God exists, moral behavior is confined. To attain *autonomous freedom*, God must die with every vestige wiped clean. This is the heart of the cultural battle in our midst, the battle for America's soul.

Existentialism: In Search of Meaning Without a God
Truth is what is True for Me

The Renaissance isolated Christianity from its foundations as men like da Vinci and Descartes began thought with the *particulars* rather than the *universals*. Enlightenment thinkers such as Voltaire and Rousseau destroyed the foundations of Christianity by separating faith and Reason, drawing an impenetrable line between the upper and lower stories. Nietzsche slew the dragon and with Existential thought, its golden "Thou Shalts" were melted and forged into the imaginings of man. What were these existential imaginings? For Karl Jaspers (1883-1969) it was the "final experience." For Jean-Paul Sartre (1905-1980) it was "self authentication." For Aldous Huxley (1894-1963) it was finding the "truth within" through the power of psychoactive drugs. *Man must have meaning—even if it is an illusion.*

The central feature of existential thought is the individual creates the meaning for his or her own existence. However, when personal belief becomes the basis of life's "*universals*," two things happen: "*universals*" are no longer universal, and "*universals*" are no longer rational. By separating the universals from Reason, Kierkegaard resurrected Siger of Brabant and the Double Mind of Man. Everyone was free to do what was right in his or her own mind. Law became law unto itself as its foundations were stripped away. "Values" became nothing more than personal preferences. Moral relativity became the accepted standard of culture. Absent a moral absolute, no Truth remained to separate one idea from another.

For example, the "final experience" existential philosopher Karl Jaspers described could not be sought, prepared for, or even communicated to another person. Yet

> *Where it is acknowledged that God exists, moral behavior is confined. To attain autonomous freedom, God must die with every vestige wiped clean. This is the heart of the cultural battle in our midst, the battle for America's soul.*

it provided the "meaning of life" for the person who had it. Existentialist Jean-Paul Sartre believed meaning is found in personally authenticating one's self through action, though one action is neither better nor worse than another. According to Sartre, there is no moral distinction between helping an elderly woman across the street and robbing her. In either case, one had "authenticated" oneself. This provides insight into his understanding that *no finite point has any meaning unless it has an infinite point of reference*. Sarte had no such point of reference, leaving him to conclude that we live in an absurd universe.

A third existentialist, Aldous Huxley, suggested giving people psychoactive medications to find "truth" within their own minds. For Huxley, "truth" was indistinguishable from a trip with LSD. With these ideas culture stumbled into profound non-Reason. It was impossible to determine societal values or maintain social mores.

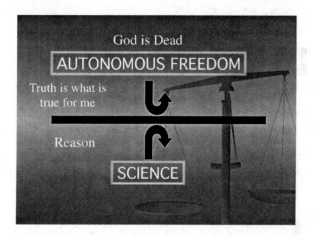

In these examples we find that by the mid-twentieth century, humanism had completely separated the *universals* from Reason. Where Thomas Aquinas and Leonardo da Vinci had struggled to find *unity* between the *particulars* and the *universals*, philosophers now eliminated the possibility of rational *universals* altogether. Even more, they exalted in their *autonomous freedom*. Here, we finally find the foundations of postmodern thought.

Recall that Voltaire's Age of Reason left man without meaning as determinism reduced him to an insignificant cog on a cosmic wheel. Postmodern thought was the final result. Man could not live without meaning—even if that meaning was just an illusion. With the Jaspers, Sartre, and Huxley, meaning became absurd as everyone defined her or her own "truth." With postmodern thought, man died a second death. Schaeffer concludes:

> No one in all the history of humanistic, rationalistic thought has found a solution [to generate meaning from himself alone]. As a result, either the thinker must say man is dead, because personality is a mirage; or else he must hang his reason on a hook outside the door and cross the threshold into the leap of faith which is the new level of despair.
>
> A man like Sir Julian Huxley has clarified the dilemma by acknowledging, though he is an atheist, that somehow or other, against all that one might expect, man functions better if he acts as though God is there. This might sound like a feasible solution for a moment, the kind of answer a computer might give if you fed the sociological data into it. God is dead, but act as if He were alive. However, a moment's reflection will show what a terrible solution this is. Isben, the Norwegian, put it like this: if you take away a man's lie, you take away his hope. These thinkers are saying in effect that man can only function as man for an extended period of time if he acts on the assumption that a lie (that the personal God of Christianity is there) is true. You cannot find any deeper despair than this...[9]

This insight of atheist Julian Huxley's is truly remarkable—"*somehow or other, against all that one might expect, man functions better if he acts as though God is there.*" This begs the response, "perhaps He is." But if this were true, the consequences would be titanic—man would no longer be the measure of all things; he could no longer create his own *universals*. If God did exist there might be a fixed moral code. For the secular humanist this is unthinkable, something that simply could not be tolerated. Postmodern thinkers would rather withhold all judgment, forsaking even the ability to condemn cannibalism, than submit to a higher moral law. Nietzsche raged against the possibility of this restraint. He was determined to sail on a sea without a shore.

Thus Have We Made the World

As history rushes down the canyon of the ages, the path it finds is hewn by the minds of men. Worldviews inexorably lead to their logical conclusions regardless of the century. History now asks, "What worldview will America choose to follow?"

While the influence of post-Enlightenment thought worked its way through Europe, a similar process reshaped society on this side of the Atlantic, only more slowly and hidden from view. America's ivory towers of academia systematically expelled God from the classroom. Medicine unwittingly gravitated toward Plato by considering euthanasia and infanticide. Law forsook her roots when the Supreme Court found the right of government to seize private property within the Fifth Amendment.

A century after the death of Nietzsche, America finds herself hovering at the edge of autonomous freedom, contemplating the once unthinkable. With all the fiery passion of Nietzsche, the secular progressive movement and postmodern thought look to destroy our country's Judeo-Christian heritage. However, in doing so, they may dismantle the very foundations of freedom.

Notes

1   Friedrich Nietzsche, *Twilight of the Idols*, p. 97.
2   Ibid., p. 99.
3   Ibid., pp. 117-118.
4   Plato, *The Republic*, translated by Benjamin Jowett, (New York: Barnes & Noble Books, 1999), p. 93.
5   Plato, *Republic*, by Waterfield, 409e-410a, p. 111.
6   Benno Muller-Hill, *Murderous Science*, (United States: Cold Spring Harbor Laboratory Press, 1998), pp. 7-22.
7   Claude J. Letulle, "Nazi Medical Experiments," United States Holocaust Memorial Museum. http://www.ushmm.org
8   Fyodor Dostoevsky, *The Brothers Karamazov*, translated by Canstance Garnett, (United States, Barnes & Noble Books, 1995), pp. xi, 60, 242, 554, 557, 593, 609.
9   Schaeffer, *Volume 1: The God Who Is There*, p. 95.

CHAPTER TWELVE

BATTLE OF WORLDVIEWS

*To challenge Darwinian theory is strictly prohibited. Why? To acknowledge
the possibility that God may actually exist is to jeopardize
Nietzsche's autonomous freedom.
This can never happen.*

The thinking of Thomas Aquinas divided history into parallel rivers of thought that thundered down the canyon of the ages. Northern and southern Europe embraced opposing solutions to answer the widespread abuse of power in the medieval church. However, as the world grew ever smaller under the weight of technology, these rivers were destined to collide. And so they did. America's present culture war reveals the explosive energy released as two diametrically opposed worldviews come crashing together. Each worldview struggles for authority; each worldview claims rightful dominance. In short, we now face the battle of "the grand sez who?"

The assumptions behind these competing worldviews (there is a higher "universal Truth" which limits human behavior vs. we create "Truth" for ourselves) are mutually exclusive, mixing with the predictable volatility of fire and gasoline. Throughout history confrontations of these worldviews repeatedly ended in death. Under the Third Reich Jews faced ovens and mass graves. In the former Soviet Republic death camps and gulags swallowed men such as Alexander Solzhenitsyn by the millions without hesitation.

Behind these atrocities lay certain commonalities in thought. We must understand the unifying threads woven throughout the tapestry of the past if we are to face the danger posed by the battle of worldviews in the present. Only then can we avoid similar travesties in the decades to come. Is this simply rhetoric? Unfortunately, history teaches us otherwise. This past century witnessed the slaughter of more innocents that any previous era, and history provides the only lens with which we can view the future.

Three concepts lie at the foundation of our modern culture war: <u>ontology</u>, <u>naturalistic</u> <u>materialism</u>, and <u>postmodern</u> <u>thought</u>. Without understanding these three necessarily difficult concepts, it is impossible to recognize the forces driving our cultural divide. Whether we turn to healthcare, the courts, education, or politics, this same battle of worldviews reappears. The reader must fully understand the information presented in this chapter and the next because it underscores all thought and Reason. Many readers may need to review this material a second time but their effort will be rewarded in the end. Without understanding how people think, it is impossible to unravel the apparent insanity of current events. *For as we think, so we are.*

Whether approaching bioethical dilemmas such as physician-assisted suicide or determining which values the Supreme Court should uphold, each individual brings his or her particular *worldview* to the table. Behind each *worldview* lies certain heuristic assumptions—assumptions that are not independently provable but are necessary for all Reason thereafter. These First Principles are the concepts we accept as true without proof before logic begins. Without exception, everyone has them.

Perhaps the single most destructive error of contemporary western thought is failing to identify our First Principles, and worse, not realizing they even exist. When the significance of First Principles is forgotten, we cannot critique our conclusions in the light of these initial assumptions. The ability to recognize errant thought is lost and eventually Reason itself is destroyed.

ONTOLOGY: AND THAT'S JUST THE WAY IT IS

Ontology is the branch of metaphysics that studies the nature of being or reality. It refers to reality as it is, not as we understand it or wish it to be.

Simply because one is unaware of something, the ontological non-existence of that particular entity does not necessarily follow. For example, the dwarf planet Pluto existed long before its discovery in 1930. Prior to that time science's lack of knowledge by no means suggests Pluto did not exist. Conversely, simply believing something is true does not make it so. For millennia people believed the Earth was flat. However, no matter how many intellectuals accepted this "fact," ontologically, it simply was not true. Public opinion, even among the elite, could never transform the Earth into a giant pancake. Ontology refers to what is, not our perception, desire, or understanding.

Understanding the concept of ontology is particularly important when it comes to answering life's ultimate questions. At the beginning of this book we explored the question "Does Truth exist or do we create 'truth' for ourselves?" This is really a formulation of a more fundamental question, "What is the origin of man?" How we answer the second question determines how we answer the first. If man is the chance product of a blind evolutionary process, there is no higher moral law. Things simply are. What is, is right. What "should be" becomes irrelevant. On the other hand, if a God created man through intelligent design, the possibility of a higher moral code exists. History offers only these two alternatives; there is no third option. The implications of which view one takes are profound.

Men such as Hooker, Rutherford, Locke, and Blackstone believed an ontologically real God (a God who really does exist) laid down limits for civil law. Recall Hooker's statement, "Human laws... also [have] higher rules to be measured by, which rules are two, the law of God, and the law of nature; so that laws human must be made according to the general laws of nature, and without contradiction to any positive law of scripture, otherwise they are ill made."[1] If these men were correct and God is indeed real, to ignore this reality would lead to the loss of all moral absolutes and eventually, to chaos. However, if Voltaire and Rousseau were correct—that God was a creation of man's imagination—to base life and civil law on such a superstition epitomized the height of irrationality. For the enlightened mind, Reason must look elsewhere—Reason must look to man.

Decisions About God's Existence Determine Our Worldview

The heuristic assumptions of Hooker and Voltaire are mutually exclusive. Ontologically speaking, theism and atheism cannot both be true. In ultimate reality, just as the dwarf planet of Pluto must either exist or not exist, God must either exist or not exist. Our personal knowledge, opinion, or desire has little to do with it. Holding to the principle of non-contradiction, a basic tenet of Aristotelian logic, God cannot both be and not be at the same time. However, there is a complicating factor. Where science unequivocally demonstrated the reality of Pluto, science will never unequivocally prove nor disprove the reality of God. Science studies phenomena of the natural world; by definition, the supernatural lies beyond the long arm of science. The question of God's existence moves beyond science into philosophy. The common misunderstanding understanding of this point drives our culture war.

The existence or non-existence of God is the First Principle on which all logic turns because it defines the foundation of our physical/material world. This assumption influences every conclusion we draw because it is the First Principle underlying every worldview. If a particular classification of ideas is defined as "unreal" or "imaginary" at the beginning, it will never receive thoughtful consideration thereafter.

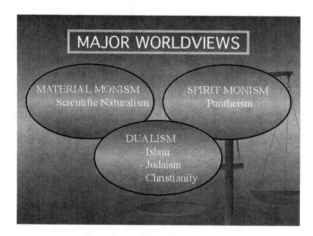

Ontologically speaking, nearly all *worldviews* can be placed in one of three categories based upon what is considered "real." In the worldview of <u>material monism</u> only the natural/physical realm is "real." By definition, nothing can exist outside the physical realm; the supernatural is a myth. Scientific naturalism falls under this category.

The worldview of <u>spirit monism</u>, on the other hand, takes precisely the opposite view of reality. Only the supernatural/spiritual realm exists and the entire experiential world is just an illusion. Pantheism (in rare forms) falls under this category. Rarely does one meet a person who truly believes this. Everyone I know uses the door when leaving a room rather than attempting to walk through the wall. The physical world is hard to deny.

A third worldview, <u>dualism</u>, combines the first two—both the natural world and the supernatural world exist in true reality. (Of note, dualism more commonly refers to the two coequal supernatural forces of good and evil. For reasons beyond the scope of this chapter, this worldview is insufficient and will not be discussed. I will use the word dualism as defined above—both the natural and the supernatural exist in true, ontological reality.) Worldviews such as Judaism, Islam, Christianity, fall under the category of dualism.

Using this construct, one begins to see that at the heart of many culturally divisive issues lay mutually exclusive First Principles. If one begins with a dualistic worldview, as did Richard Hooker, Samuel Rutherford, and the great majority of America's Founding Fathers, not only is the acceptance of a higher moral law possible, it is perfectly rational. In fact, if these men are correct, the rejection of this reality becomes irrational.

Nearly all worldviews can be placed in one of three categories based upon what is considered "real."

However, if one begins with the worldview of naturalism, as did the Enlightenment thinkers Voltaire and Rousseau, precisely the opposite is true. If God does not exist in ontological reality, man is left to make law for himself. To appeal to a higher moral code is irrational, nothing more than superstition used as a tool to control the masses.

In this battle of worldviews, we are back to the division between the northern and southern European thought.

SCIENTIFIC NATURALISM: A MOTHERLESS MOTHER NATURE

The material monistic worldview of <u>scientific naturalism</u> goes by many names. It is most properly called *naturalistic materialism*—a purely *natural* process produced the *material* world that we know. Sometimes it is called <u>naturalism</u>, or even more simply, <u>materialism</u>. This worldview is closely tied to the <u>secular progressive movement</u>; however, this phrase refers to the social/ political effort seeking to implement the logical conclusions of the worldview of scientific naturalism.

In the previous diagram the supernatural does not exist within the upper left oval, only the material world is believed to exist in ontological reality. Within this worldview choosing to believe in God for personal reasons is fine (many materialists do), but one cannot credibly claim that God actually exists and is involved with earthly affairs. (Recall Siger of Brabant: He thought the church needed to be correct theologically, but it was permissible to be wrong scientifically. In turn, the scientist could think Christianity was nonsense but he or she could believe that Christianity held some meaning at a personal level, even if it was nonsense scientifically.) By definition God and the supernatural are fictional. To believe otherwise is irrational—the antithesis of Reason. These assumptions determine the logical conclusions of this worldview.

Naturalism: The Assumption of Post-Darwinian Science

Modern science now operates exclusively within a naturalistic worldview, a position justified in at least two ways. First, assuming the material world is the result of a natural process pushes scientific understanding onward. Excluding supernatural possibilities compels science to continue looking for ever-better natural explanations. Without this assumption seemingly unknowable phenomena might be left with only a mystical explanation. Recall Aristotle's Prime Mover, the outermost crystalline sphere that propelled planetary motion. This imaginary view stood for nearly two millennia. Only when Copernicus, Galileo, Kepler, and Newton replaced Aristotle's theory with scientific experimentation based on physics and mathematics, did we gain an accurate understanding of the cosmos. For modern science, leaving mystical explanations in place is unacceptable.

Second, scientific naturalism appears to be a necessary assumption. The scientific method of hypothesis, experimentation, and observation assumes cause and effect. More precisely it assumes natural cause and effect and gives heavy weight to reproducibility. If the supernatural did exist, it would be neither controllable nor reproducible making it impossible to study from a scientific vantage point. In fact the meaning of the Latin root, *supernaturalis*, "above nature," tells the story. Because science operates exclusively within the natural realm, it is impossible to know when forces "above nature" are at work or when a natural process is simply not understood. The cleanest approach is to simply exclude the possibility of the supernatural at the outset. This is what science currently does.

However, we must remember that early scientists did not find it necessary to take this view. The early scientists who displaced Aristotle's imaginary Prime Mover believed that to understand nature was to understand God. For men such as Copernicus, Kepler, and Galileo, believing that a rational God created a rational universe provided the expectation that science was possible. Yet they still expected the natural world to work naturally. The story of Galileo's repeated dropping of an iron ball from the Leaning Tower of Pisa recording the time it took to fall demonstrates an expectation that each subsequent drop of the ball to follow in a fashion similar to the first. He did not expect the last ball dropped to stop three feet above the ground, levitate for an extra five seconds, then finish falling.

In the wake of the Enlightenment this formulation changed. Voltaire, Rousseau, and others embraced a naturalistic worldview based upon the understanding that man created God, not the other way around. When this worldview captured the minds of scientists during the mid-nineteenth century, the search for a natural explanation of the origin of life was on. *If God did not exist, there must be a natural explanation for the existence of life, there was no other possibility*. This philosophy permeated scientific thought throughout Europe when Darwin published *The Origin of Species* in 1859. Given the overwhelming success of physics, biology, and chemistry, science was unwilling accept theistic explanations for the origin of man. From the naturalist's perspective, to give up on a natural explanation for the origin of life was to give up on science itself.

Almost overnight Darwinian thought became a fundamental law of science. Soon, to challenge Darwin's theory was to challenge the scientific method itself. This is understandable in context of worldviews. If one begins within the upper left circle of material monism, a theory appealing to anything other than a purely natural process is mythical (wrong) by definition.

Here we must take a moment to differentiate between two types of knowledge. The first is *a priori* knowledge—knowledge accepted as Truth *prior to* examination of the evidence. *A priori* knowledge is a First Principle, a heuristic assumption accepted as true *before* Reason begins; it is not based upon scientific investigation. A second type of knowledge is *a posteriori* knowledge—knowledge gained *after* examination of the evidence. *A posteriori* knowledge is what science seeks to achieve through experimentation and observation. A brief story portrays the importance of distinguishing between these two types of knowledge.

Darwinism and the Two Types of Knowledge

In his book *Darwin on Trial*, Phillip Johnson recounts a fascinating story contrasting these two types of knowledge as applied to the theory of evolution. The 1967 Philadelphia Wistar Institute Conference examining the probability of Darwinian evolution reveals that modern science accepts Darwinian thought as *a priori* knowledge (something known *before* examination of the facts), not solely as a conclusion based upon compelling evidence.

At this particular conference a mathematician named D. S. Ulam argued that Darwinian evolution (the steady accumulation of numerous small mutations) of the eye was highly improbable—the number of mutations needed was far too large for the time allowed by the fossil record. In response, Sir Peter Medawar and C. H. Waddington asserted Ulam had it backwards; because the eye *had* evolved the mathematical difficulties were only apparent, not real. Another Darwinist, Ernst Mayr, concluded, "Somehow or other by adjusting these figures we will come out all right. We are confronted by the fact that evolution has occurred."[2]

Even though the Darwinists and the mathematicians both rejected intelligent design as a possibility (a theory that can exist only in a dualistic worldview), it is important to recognize the *type* of logic each employed. Ulam used *a posteriori* reasoning. He looked at the mathematical evidence *and then* formulated his conclusion—in light of his findings he doubted the Darwinian model was plausible. If the Darwinists likewise used *a posteriori* reasoning, Ulam's point needed further exploration. Had he miscalculated? Had he made valid assumptions? If Ulam's research was valid, Darwin's theory needed reworking.

However, the Darwinists accepted evolution as fact *a priori* (knowledge accepted as Truth *before* examination of the evidence). Using this reasoning, Ulam *must* be wrong—not because his research was flawed, but simply because he called Darwin into question. As Johnson succinctly states, for Darwinists, Darwinism "was not a theory open to refutation but a fact to be accounted for."[3]

Notice what transpired here. The philosophy of science changed. Rather than being open to wherever scientific inquiry led, conclusions were now dictated by a naturalistic worldview.

Notice what transpired here. The *philosophy of science* changed. Rather than being open to scientific inquiry—wherever it led—conclusions were now dictated by a naturalistic worldview. The *a priori* philosophical assumption of naturalistic materialism—the *worldview*—was now the undisputable filter through which all evidence passed. Evidence supporting Darwin was "science," evidence to the contrary was discarded. *Scientific conclusions were not based upon academic rigor but upon the worldview reinforced.* (The same is now true for much of the mainstream media, but that is a subject for another book.) This filter of worldviews exerts its influence at multiple levels within the academic community, of which we will briefly examine three.

Three Examples of how Modern Academia Excludes the Dualistic Worldview

1) The scientific community's active exclusion of everything outside the naturalistic worldview by was portrayed in late 2004. On August 4th a serious, peer-reviewed scientific journal published a paper by Stephen Meyer calling Darwinian theory into question and arguing instead for intelligent design. Richard Sternberg, the managing editor responsible for Meyer's paper

being published, received immediate criticism. Even though Sternberg held two PhD's (one in molecular evolution and a second in systems science) and was a Staff Scientist at the Smithsonian Institute, his credentials came under assault. The publisher repudiated the paper and reaffirmed its commitment to Darwinian thought the following month.

According to Sternberg, the Smithsonian Institute then aggressively sought to have him removed. Finding no legal grounds to fire him, he was deprived of workspace, transferred to a hostile supervisor, not allowed access to research materials, and forced to relinquish his master key. On several occasions the Smithsonian pressured him (against the ethical standards of academic publishing) to reveal the names of the three scientists who reviewed the paper and repeatedly told him that he should have found reviewers who would have rejected the paper outright.[4] Clearly the Smithsonian Institute did not believe the rules of academic freedom applied to those holding a dualistic worldview.

2) A second example is the case of Dean Kenyon, Professor Emeritus of biology at San Francisco State University. In 1969 Kenyon coauthored *Biochemical Predestination*, a standard book on the evolutionary origins of life. Despite his numerous academic achievements, Kenyon became embroiled in controversy when he became convinced traditional Darwinian theory was insufficient.

By 1980 Kenyon regularly discussed shortcomings of Darwin's theory in his introductory biology class. Along with these doubts he presented alternative positions, including intelligent design. In 1992 a handful of students complained about this practice. The department chair censured Kenyon and subsequently removed him as course instructor. Kenyon appealed to the faculty's Academic Freedom Committee. As a senior professor, he maintained part of his academic responsibility was to make students aware of shortcomings of any particular theory and present alternate views. In this case, the Academic Freedom Committee agreed and Kenyon was reinstated. But as with the Richard Sternberg/Smithsonian Institute case, the attempt to suppress evidence that questioned Darwinian thought was clear.

3) John Searle provides a third example. As a committed naturalist and professor of philosophy at University of California, Berkeley, Searle takes this process to the extreme. Searle not only refuses to debate the possibility of intelligent design, Searle eliminates the vocabulary of those holding a dualistic worldview rendering them unable to even articulate a rebuttal. In his book *Mind, Language, and Society* he states:

> The result of this demystification is that we have gone beyond atheism to the point where the issue no longer matters in the way it did to earlier generations. For us, if it should turn out that God exists, that would have to be a fact of nature like any other.... If the supernatural existed, it too would have to be natural.[5]

Pause to note what just happened. Here we find a passion rivaling Nietzsche's will to power and a twist of logic that competes with Hegelian synthesis. Searle states, "If the supernatural existed, it too would have to be natural." He is held so captive by his materialistic worldview that he redefines the word "supernatural" to mean its opposite, "natural." This eliminates any possible resurrection of God. It is impossible to argue for a reality "above nature" because, if Searle had his way, no words would be left to even express the concept.

The materialistic worldview so permeates the academic community to question it is unthinkable. For those holding a naturalistic worldview, dualism is irrational by definition. Rather than remembering naturalistic materialism is an un-provable philosophical assumption, modern academia accepts it as the given on which all else is built. In each of these examples science no longer invites debate in pursuit of Truth and understanding. Rather, it aggressively turns on all who threaten its naturalistic base. To challenge this worldview is strictly prohibited.

To challenge Darwinian theory is strictly prohibited. Why? To acknowledge the possibility that God may actually exist is to jeopardize Nietzsche's autonomous freedom. This can never happen.

Why? To acknowledge the possibility that God may actually exist is to jeopardize Nietzsche's *autonomous freedom*. This can never happen. Materialism is axiomatic.

The Initial Assumptions Determine the Conclusions

Recall that Euclid began his geometry with axioms such as "two points determine a line," and "there is one and only one line parallel to a given line through a given point." From these axioms, Euclidian geometry is logically extrapolated. It is possible to begin with different axioms; these lead to a non-Euclidean geometries, such as the geometry of spherical surface rather than a plane. Both types of geometry are the logical consequences of their initial axioms. *To determine the assumptions is to determine the conclusions if logic is applied consistently.*

Given science's presupposition of naturalistic materialism, a great deal has been explained without invoking the supernatural. Quite often, previously held mystical explanations were reversed as natural mechanistic understanding progressed. Reinforced by repeated success in understanding the natural world, the expectation developed that all things that could not be explained would eventually be elucidated if science was given enough time. This expectation then became an assumption and naturalism silently crept into the halls of scientifically proven fact.

Yet, in forgotten reality, the worldview of naturalism is not based on modern science. Rather, it is modern science that is based on naturalism. The naturalistic worldview remains the same philosophical presupposition it always has been—it remains in the upper left oval based upon the assumption that God does not exist. *Naturalistic materialism is a philosophy.* Ontologically, it holds no more weight than intelligent design—the philosophical presupposition held by those who begin with a dualistic worldview. The non-existence of God never has been, and never will be proven by the scientific method. By definition the supernatural lies beyond nature in a world that science cannot explore.

However, the general public does not understand this. *When academia positioned Darwinism as a scientifically proven fact, the naturalistic worldview followed it into the classroom uncontested. By definition it was the only rational conclusion. Darwinism was used to prove naturalistic materialism when, in fact,*

212

Darwinism was the only possible alternative when one began with a materialistic worldview.

THE AGGRESSIVE DEFENSE OF DARWIN

The hostility directed at Sternberg and Kenyon betrays the social implications in the battle for the soul of science. Science is no longer pure science; it has become a philosophy. This shift lies at the heart of our culture war. Sternberg violated a sacred secret when he published a peer-reviewed scientific paper challenging the supremacy of Darwinism. Why did this evoke such opposition? Because of the social implications.

If Darwin goes, so does the philosophical and intellectual foundation of modern liberal thought. Recall the words of Richard Dawkins, "Darwin made it possible to be an intellectually fulfilled atheist."[6] Darwin "proved" that God was unnecessary granting man *autonomous freedom*. Every ounce of passion that Nietzsche used to kill God will rise once again to defend Darwin. If Darwin was wrong, then God might exist. If God exists, then man is not autonomous. And for those who follow in the footsteps of Nietzsche the possibility of man losing autonomous freedom is unthinkable.

Ironically, by suppressing the theory of intelligent design, "science" and modern liberalism are doing precisely what classical liberalism raged against—they are censoring critical thought and the free expression of competing ideas. At first glance this appears self-contradictory, however, if we understand the underlying worldview it makes perfect sense.

Classical liberalism passionately championed the basic human freedoms our Founding Fathers believed were endowed on us by our Creator: the freedom of speech, the freedom of association, the freedom of religion, and the private ownership of property. Modern liberalism is bent on *autonomous freedom*, destroying anything that stands in the way.

Modern liberalism not only owns academia, it understands autonomous freedom rises and falls with Darwin. It also understands that if intelligent

> Science is no longer pure science; it has become a philosophy. Sternberg violated a sacred secret when he published a peer-reviewed scientific paper challenging the supremacy of Darwinism. Why did this evoke such opposition? Because of the social implications. If Darwin goes, so does the philosophical and intellectual foundation of modern liberal thought.

design gained a platform to make its case, Darwin's hegemony would end. Academia now uses its influence and the courts to ensure this debate never takes place.

In the introduction to his book *Reason in the Balance*, former Supreme Court clerk and current Berkeley law professor Phillip Johnson offers a concise description of the mindset in academia. Paraphrasing him closely: *The secularist argues that naturalism reigns in academia because naturalism is based upon science; intelligent design is based upon religion. Science uses Reason based upon knowledge. Religion only provides belief based upon faith. Science, reason, and knowledge trump religion, faith, and belief every time.*[7] Therefore public education teaches *naturalism* as science and excludes *intelligent design* as belief.

The error of this argument, of course, is the premise. *Naturalism* is not built on science; it is a philosophy—a worldview. Conversely, science is now built on *naturalism*, a philosophical assumption that may be wrong. *If the assumption is wrong, the conclusions will be wrong as well.* America has confused what science has proven with the philosophical assumptions science makes before even taking its first step down the road of discovery.

Wrong Assumptions Lead to Wrong Conclusions

While modern scientific experimentation has good reason to argue for the working presupposition of *naturalism*, this position has one major shortcoming—*it may not be true.* The possibility remains that an ontologically real supernatural does exist and can intervene in the human experience. This is the other equally valid working presupposition (the null-hypothesis of *naturalistic materialism*). To forget this is to blind oneself to a possibility that, if true, would bring one to a completely different set of conclusions when looking at the same data. To ignore this possibility, as science presently does, is actually *unscientific.* It excludes a potential influencing factor without consideration, thus biasing the observers' conclusions.

For the sake of argument let us accept the possibility that the universe did come into being through intelligent design. If science begins with a worldview of naturalism then no matter what the evidence reveals, modern science will never reach the correct conclusion. A more expansive view would be to acknowledge both sets of philosophical presuppositions (naturalism and theism), perform the experimentation, *and then determine which bests fits observed data*. However, in my 15 years of formal scientific education, I never saw this done.

It is tragic, yet fascinating, to watch this story unfold. As noted earlier, even non-Christian scholar and prominent physicist Robert Oppenheimer concluded it was the Christian worldview that gave us modern science—an orderly God created an orderly universe that could be understood. Yet we find the present philosophy of modern science excludes the possibility of a real God from meaningful consideration. Science killed the very worldview that gave it birth.

Modern science (as a naturalistic philosophy, not as the scientific method of hypothesis/null hypothesis properly understood) has also killed our source of personality and individual worth. Time, chance, and Darwinian selection pressure are *non-personal* forces. These stand in contrast to the Judeo-Christian worldview of intelligent design by a *personal* God. How personality and individuality arise from a non-personal source has never been shown. Yet, even though science has removed a rational source of true personality, culture finds it anyway. Western culture now refers to the cold, purposeless process of evolution as "Mother Nature." Irrationally, we inject personality into a non-personal process. This begs the question, "Why?" Could it be we *are* personal beings craving individual worth?

These concepts of metaphysics may appear too esoteric and bothersome to worry about understanding—a mere straining at gnats—but nothing could be more dangerous to America than to think this. Naturalism has not only washed away the foundations of human dignity but the foundations for the rule of law as well. And the ramifications of this mistake are profound.

Notes

1   John Locke quoting Richard Hooker, *Second Treatise of Government*, (Indianapolis Indiana: Hackett Publishing Company, 1980), p. 71.

2   Phillip Johnson, *Darwin On Trial*, (Downers Grove, Illinois: Intervarsity Press, 1993), pp. 38, 39.

3   Ibid., p. 39.

4   Richard Sterberg, www.rsternberg.net/index.htm,

5   John Searle, *Mind, Language, and Society*, (New York: BasicBooks, 1998), p. 35.
6   Richard Dawkins, *The Blind Watchmaker*, (New York: W.W.Norton & Company, 1996), p. 6.
7   Phillip Johnson, *Reason in the Balance*, (Downers Grove, Illinois: Intervarsity Press, 1995), p 10.

CHAPTER THIRTEEN

MAN AS A MACHINE: PERSONALITY IS DESTROYED

Unless you assume a God, the question
of life's purpose is meaningless.
Bertrand Russell, atheist (1872-1970)

Academia defends Darwin's Theory with such passion because it provides the philosophical base for autonomous freedom. If Darwin falls, autonomous freedom falls with it and a postmodern world can never let this happen. However, Darwin's thought carries a significant unintended consequence—in the wake of Darwinian philosophy, man becomes a machine.

The worldviews of *naturalistic materialism* and Judeo-Christianity come head to head over what it means to be human. What it means to be human flows directly from the heuristic assumptions made about the existence or non-existence of God—the First Principle behind all bioethical thought. Here, two alternatives confront us.

First, the phenomenon of complex life-forms appearing in a purely naturalistic universe is best explained using the "Blind Watchmaker Theory," a phrase taken from the book by Richard Dawkins, *The Blind Watchmaker.*[1] Dawkins, professor at Oxford University, is perhaps the world's most prominent Darwinist and his book is a classic in the Darwinian canon. In this theory, mankind evolved from vastly lower life forms—even non-life forms—simply with the passage of time, chance, and Darwinian selection pressure. The driving force behind this theory is the accumulation of beneficial mutations. The vast majority of mutations are damaging to the organism making them less fit to survive. These organisms die early and are removed from the gene pool. The few remaining beneficial mutations are naturally selected for and retained. Given time the beneficial mutations accumulate and new species emerge. The Blind Watchmaker Theory asserts man is the result of a random process without planning, purpose, or the influence of an intelligent being.

The philosophical counter to this is known as *intelligent design*, perhaps most articulately argued by former Supreme Court clerk and Berkeley law professor, Phillip Johnson.[2] Johnson does not argue for a seven day Genesis literalism but asserts only intelligence can account for the genetic complexity required for life. The Judeo-Christian worldview offers such an intelligent Being.

When comparing these two *worldviews* (the way we view the world around us based on our assumptions about ultimate reality), examining the evidence for and against each perspective would seem a logical place to begin. However, evidence is proof only to those who wish to see it as proof. Each side reviews and sanctions the facts that support its position, wondering why opponents cannot see the obvious. Each explains away and discounts the evidence that brings its own position into question. At the end of the day, there is a stalemate. Few are moved even to an understanding of the other's point of view. Another approach is to examine their logical conclusions.

The Meaning of Man

Within the Judeo-Christian worldview (as set forth by Iraneus, St. Augustine, and Thomas Aquinas) we find the concept of the *Imago Dei*. This provides intrinsic dignity to the human by claiming humanity was fashioned to bear the image of God. A real and personal God intentionally designed a real and personal being distinct from the rest of the animal kingdom. The *Imago Dei* infused humanity with intrinsic value, meaning, and purpose. Until recently, this has been a core assumption of medical ethics. Even for

Hippocrates the basis for the sanctity of human life emanated from religious conviction, from a source of moral authority higher than man.

The intrinsic value of human life for those holding this worldview stands in stark contrast to the devaluation of human life for those who follow Darwin. Accepting the view of *naturalistic materialism* makes God obsolete. It does not pronounce God dead as Nietzsche did, but rather removes God from meaningful consideration, making Him immaterial in both uses of the word. If God is inconsequential, no higher moral authority remains to impute innate moral value to human life. The ramifications of a culture's transition from a Judeo-Christian worldview to naturalism are monumental. Quotes from three prominent naturalists best explain this position.

First, historian Carl Becker in a series of lectures at Yale Law School in 1931 noted:

> Edit and interpret the conclusions of modern science as tenderly as we like, it is still quite impossible for us to regard man as the child of God for whom the earth was created as a temporary habitation. Rather must we regard him as little more than a chance deposit on the surface of the world, carelessly thrown up between two ice ages by the same forces that rust iron and ripen corn...[3,4]

Second, biologist George Gaylord Simpson in *The Meaning of Evolution* published in 1949 stated:

> Although many details remain to be worked out, it is already evident that all the objective phenomena of the history of life can be explained by purely naturalistic or, in a proper sense of the sometimes abused word, materialistic factors... Man is the result of a purposeless and natural process that did not have him in mind.[5]

The third is Francis Crick, recipient of the Nobel Peace Prize in 1962 along with James Watson for discovering the double stranded helix of DNA:

> [Y]our joys and your sorrows, your memories and your
> ambitions, your sense of personal identity and free will, are
> in fact no more than the behavior of a vast assembly of nerve
> cells and their associated molecules.[6]

These represent hundreds of similar quotations. For all three men life is meaningless. Given this worldview, even love, one of life's most wonderful and intense emotions, becomes only the firing of neurons. Pleasurable as it may be, it is of no higher value than hate—neurons fire and release their associated neurotransmitters no matter the emotion. The human experience is a mere winding down of Newton's clocklike universe. Nothing awaits man but a cold, still end, no different than a stalk of rotting corn. The difficulty is humans *inwardly know* something separates them from a hunk of rusting iron.

Only a personal being can produce personality. Personality cannot arise from a random, non-personal process. Furthermore, personality is the basis of human individuality. If we are really the outcome of a random, non-intelligent, non-personal process, "little more than a chance deposit on the surface of the world, carelessly thrown up between two ice ages by the same forces that rust iron and ripen corn," the illusion of personality/individuality becomes a cruel joke. If in ontological reality we are inconsequential, non-personal beings thrown up by a meaningless, random process, to feel at the center of our being that we are unique individuals with intrinsic dignity is no more than a cheap trick of a motherless nature.

Man as a Machine, What is, is Right

Marquis de Sade (1740-1814) believed that man was determined, the end product of an uncaring, purposeless process. Given this worldview, de Sade believed what is, is right. There is no higher purpose; there is no higher law. He applied this worldview to sexual morality. Nature generally made men stronger than women. Because this is the natural order of things, in his mind there is nothing wrong with a man beating his wife for pleasure. It is the logical result of nature. As he wrote in *La Nouvelle Justine*, "As nature has made us [the men] the strongest, we can do with her [the women] whatever we please."[7]

We get our word *sadism* from Marquis de Sade. At its root, sadism in not simply inducing pain for sexual pleasure, it represents an irrefutable conclusion of *naturalism*. "What is, is right." Man is a machine devoid of meaning and devoid of morality. To take the position that anything is morally wrong is irrational. Beginning with *naturalism*, it is impossible to rationally argue against de Sade.

The *naturalist* can describe "what is" with great detail, but cannot determine "what is good." A random process cannot produce a moral outcome. Even the assumption that something is good because it preserves human life has no logical base (though personally, humans find this concept very convenient). Some would argue that the Earth would be better with humanity's extinction because humans are the only species capable of destroying nature. But this argument is based on the assumption that it is good for nature to continue to exist undisturbed, which again is inconsistent with the *worldview* of naturalism. "What is, is right," even if "what is" is the end of nature. Beginning with naturalist presuppositions, to argue otherwise is irrational. When isolated from the *universals*, Reason inexorably leads us into a world without meaning, into a world in which we cannot live.

> *"What is, is right,"* even if it is the end of nature... When isolated from the universals, Reason inexorably leads us into a world without meaning, into a world in which we cannot live.

Operating within the worldview of naturalism, academia now declares God and religion irrational. Beginning with naturalist presuppositions, American courts have stripped nearly all of Christianity's influence from public schools leaving our children to believe they are the end products of a random and purposeless process. Yet somehow, we irrationally expect morality, dignity, and honor to survive.

Why the surprise at rising school violence? Students are only living out the *worldview* they have been taught. Human life is not special. There are no rational boundaries. In Carl Becker's words, human life is "little more than a chance deposit on the surface of the world, carelessly thrown up between two ice ages by the same forces that rust iron and ripen corn." If "what is, is right," why not act with reckless abandon?

But what of the possibility that humans crave meaning because, ontologically, *life has meaning*? What of the possibility that high school

...... college students go to extremes to find individuality because *they are individuals with true personality.* When reared in a world without moral boundaries and educated under a system that continually teaches that life has no ultimate purpose, the logical end is intense frustration. There is no limit to the insanity that will follow.

In 1998 Peter Singer was appointed to the Ira W. DeCamp Professorship of Bioethics, a prestigious endowed chair at Princeton University. In his book *Rethinking Life and Death—The collapse of Our Traditional Ethics,* he defines a new moral code.[8] In keeping with Nietzsche's child, Singer removes the concept of the *Imago Dei,* erases the Ten Commandments, annuls the principle of the sanctity of life, *then* rethinks the foundations of moral thought. Based on *naturalistic* assumptions, he lays out Five New Commandments concluding that the human fetus is morally equivalent to a rat or a fish.[9] He considers the view of humans intrinsically having greater moral value than other animals as "speciesist." These ideas sound extreme, but they need to be taken seriously. Singer received international acclaim for these views. (Ironically, Princeton's motto is *Dei Sub Numine Viget,* "Under God's Power She Flourishes."[10])

> If meaning, morals, and individuality were to be regained, they must be found by way of an irrational leap. As night follows day, the Age of Reason inescapably led to the Age of Non-Reason.

To Singer's credit, like de Sade, he remains intellectually consistent with his initial assumptions. As an avid *naturalist* he maintains that we are the products of time, chance, and Darwinian selection pressure. If each species is simply the product of a random process, there is no logical reason to claim one has more intrinsic worth than another. Though it is certainly convenient to claim that human life is special (every reader of this book is human), this position does not logically follow from the initial heuristic presuppositions of naturalism.

In contrast, personality and the intrinsic value of human life is the logical conclusion only when one begins with an ontologically real and personal God creating a real and personal being.

The logical end of *naturalism*—there is no meaning, no morality, and no individuality. Beginning with the First Principles of naturalism, Reason led humanity into a wasteland of the absurd. However, culture could not live with this. If meaning, morality, and individuality were to be regained, they must be found by way of an irrational leap. As night follows day, the Age of Reason inescapably led to the Age of Non-Reason. Modernity had no alternative but to spill over into postmodernity. And with this came the death of Truth.

POSTMODERNISM: TRUTH IS NO LONGER TRUE

Nature abhors a vacuum. When *naturalism* destroyed meaning, it destroyed dignity. Humanity hung over an abyss, grasping for anything that might forestall the terrible conclusion that man was a machine—devoid of will, robbed of autonomy. Following modernity personality and individuality were now logically impossible—they were merely illusions masking the profound emptiness of life. This abyss signaled modernism would eventually fall; man could not live with the conclusions of Marquis de Sade and the logical end of *naturalism*. Postmodern thought was inevitable.

> The genius of postmodern thought is that it appears to restore personality and individuality without threatening autonomous freedom. However, when Truth becomes what is "true for me," Truth is no more than opinion and Reason gives way to non-Reason.

Postmodernism is the inescapable conclusion of a worldview that declares God immaterial, of a worldview without a source of purpose and moral certainty. Briefly stated, premodern Western civilization understood Truth to be of supernatural origin. But Nietzsche concluded Truth could not come from God—God was dead. Modernism defined Truth as what could be proven by science. Yet a mechanical universe based on Reason erased man's dignity— man was a machine. The remaining alternative was postmodernism—Truth lay within the individual. The genius of this solution was that it appeared to restore personality and individuality without threatening autonomous freedom. However, when Truth became what is "true for me," Truth was no more than an opinion. Reason had given way to non-Reason.

While postmodern thought rejects the idea of a moral standard to which all are subject, it does not abandon the idea of moral behavior. Many postmodern thinkers are "good" and "moral" people by common usage of the words. However, they generate their own morality using an existential leap.

Much like Kierkegaard's leap of faith, postmodern morality lacks a rational tie to the underlying worldview.

Most simply defined, postmodernism asserts that there are no absolutes. The difficulty is this assertion proves itself false; it is a philosophical base standing in contradiction with itself. One can declare the concept of "right and wrong" is erroneous only by using the concept of "right and wrong." Postmodern thought assumes itself to be universally true while declaring there is no universal Truth. It states with absolute certainty that there is nothing of which we can be absolutely certain.

So the case of postmodern thought must be restated. There are no absolutes, that is, except one. *No one else* can claim an absolute. This intellectually indefensible absolute is defended with religious fervor; and then, amazingly enough, it continues to take itself seriously, deriding all who call this stunning illogic into question. This "worldview of tolerance" is tolerant only of worldviews with which it agrees. It attempts to crush any worldview that contemplates such a thing as Truth. For the concept of Truth threatens *autonomous freedom*, the pinnacle of post-Enlightenment striving.

Since the days of ancient Greece, two dominant thought forms circled each other, preparing for a final confrontation where the winner takes all. One yields to a higher moral law, the other seeks to create law for itself. They now square off, ready to battle for America's soul. Here lies our fate.

Postmodern Thought in American Culture

Postmodern thought destroys the ability to distinguish between good and evil. True postmodern thinkers are unable to say that Hitler was evil. They find it impossible to *know* America and its allies were morally justified in removing him from power. They can only go as far as to say that they could not personally do what he did, but to make a moral judgment is a greater transgression than the gas chambers of Dachau. Likewise, the postmodern thinker cannot distinguish between Saddam Hussein's longstanding human rights violations and President Bush's commitment to remove him from power and return Iraq to its people. True postmodernists reserve their condemnation only for those who claim a source of moral authority—specifically for those who hold a Judeo-Christian worldview.

Hence we see passionate outcry against President Bush for framing the Iraqi war using moral language of good and evil, certain that America is acting on the side of the good. The anger was stated in terms of the war being concocted prior to 9/11, of Bush lying to the world, betraying the American people. Such moral certainty is of greater offense than Saddam's mass graves; President Bush trespassed postmodernism's only moral law.

As American culture embraces postmodern thought, this radical alteration in the concept of Truth is fueling titanic social change. America once had a shared set of fixed values based upon a common, transcendent ethic: honesty, integrity, faithfulness, honor… A common, unspoken awareness emerged when these core values were violated. Shared values brought national unity. We saw this following Pearl Harbor. America responded with unity as people from all walks of life recognized the evil enveloping Europe and the Pacific. Whether rationing gasoline, shipbuilding, or fighting, each contributed to free Europe from despotism. During World War II most of America understood her enemy.

America now faces the battle of "the grand sez who?" The only position that is unacceptable is to say something is unacceptable. The cultural ramifications of this moral bankruptcy cannot be overstated.

However, with the advancement of postmodern thought during the past fifty years America has relinquished the moral standard with which it once made moral judgments. We have lost our ability to distinguish good from evil. "One man's solder is another man's freedom fighter." Because "Truth" resides within each individual, one idea carries no more intrinsic authority than any other. Reason itself breaks down without unifying concepts to which to appeal leaving everything open for debate. Each position is relative. Any restraint of behavior is met with fierce opposition as *autonomous freedom* reigns supreme.

America now faces the battle of "the grand sez who?" The only position that is now unacceptable is to say something is unacceptable. The cultural ramifications of this moral bankruptcy cannot be overstated.

How Postmodernism Rewrites History

The influence of postmodern thought reaches beyond the metaphysical present into the historical past. Just as "Truth" is a matter of personal opinion, history is also subject to interpretation. In his book *Postmodern Times*, Gene Edward Veith describes the dismantling of history itself:

> Postmodernists also seek to dissolve history. They no longer see it as a record of objective facts, but as "a series of metaphors which cannot be detached from the institutionally produced languages which we bring to bear on it." As a result... we can make no distinction between "truth" and "fiction." "History is a network of agonistic language games where the criterion for success is performance not truth."
>
> Since there is no objective truth, history may be rewritten according to the needs of a particular group. If history is nothing more that "a network of agonistic... language games," then any alternative "language game" that advances a particular agenda, that meets "success" in countering institutional power can pass as legitimate history.[11]

This statement is stunning. Not even history is True. It is something to mold and modify for political gain. Veith goes on to note that a whole generation of teachers, lawyers, judges, journalists, and politicians were immersed in this form of thinking while receiving their education. When even the objective Truth of history is lost, the projection of "truth" then becomes nothing more than an act of power; we have returned to Nietzsche. "Truth" is "will to power." History can be rewritten to enforce whatever position is politically expedient. Scholarship is little more than rhetorical manipulation.

During his research for the book *Original Intent*, David Barton found a startling example of this.[12] Alexis de Tocqueville's *Democracy in America* (1835) has long since been a classical observation of early American life and political climate. De Tocqueville came from France to examine and document the American experiment. He was not Christian and was not used to the integration of faith and politics. In France religion and politics were completely separated. As we have seen humanism formed the philosophical underpinnings of politics in France. Because of this background, de Tocqueville considered the close linkage of the two in America rather remarkable and wrote at some length about the interconnection between family, morality, religion, and their impact on political life in America.

Significant here is Richard D. Heffner's translation of *Democracy in America* that was "Specially Edited and Abridged for the Modern Reader."[13] It is revealing which passages he chooses to omit. For example, the following paragraphs were deleted.

> Upon my arrival in the United States, the religious aspect of the country was the first thing that struck my attention; and the longer I stayed there, the more did I perceive the great political consequences resulting from this state of things to which I was unaccustomed. In France I had almost always seen the spirit of religion and the spirit of freedom marching in pursuing courses diametrically opposed to each other; but in America, I found they were intimately united and they reigned in common over the same country.[14]

> The Americans combine the notions of Christianity and of liberty so intimately in their minds that it is impossible to make them conceive the one without the other.[15]

This is but one example of how academia selectively denies our youth a full understanding of history. Left to run its course, postmodern revisionism will rid public education of our Judeo-Christian heritage entirely. If our heritage is not taught, how will our next generation of leaders appreciate and preserve the foundations of freedom? If a non-Christian French observer recognized the clear link between our Founding Fathers' Judeo-Christian worldview and their defense of liberty, shouldn't this be taught? However, a student reading Heffner's text, "Specially Edited and Abridged for the (Post-Modern) Reader", would remain ignorant of one of de Tocqueville's most important observations. But for the postmodern, history is what we wish to make it.

The Battle Over Truth

This battle of worldviews—the battle over the concept of Truth—goes far beyond the Supreme Court decision of *Kelo v. New London*, America's healthcare policy, or how history is taught, even as profound as these are. This struggle touches every aspect of public life as it rends this country in two. In fact, it speaks to America's survival and her continued self-rule. President Barack Obama proudly claimed "world citizenship" to the roar of applause in Germany. Just as Plato surrendered the liberty of Greek citizens to the ruling elite, America contemplates yielding its position as the great defender of freedom to a world body.

Why do some people believe the United Nations or the European Union understand the foundations of freedom better than the American patriot? Why do some of America's political leaders so willingly agree to subject America to foreign control? Why do some Americans so eagerly blame our great nation only to ignore the atrocities we see overseas?

Postmodern thought (and its inability to discern good from evil) lies at the heart of these political battles. In an age of global terrorism, America must remain united to fight a common enemy. However, in the years following 9/11 America moved away from national unity toward aggressive self-destruction. Only by understanding these powerful forces that threaten to destroy our country can *we the people* avoid falling prey to the *autonomous freedom* of postmodern thought. Our greatest adversary approaches not from outside our borders, but from within.

Notes

1   Richard Dawkins, *The Blind Watchmaker: Why the evidence of Evolution Reveals a Universe Without Design*, (New York & London: W. W. Norton and Company, 1987).

2   Phillip Johnson, *Darwin On Trial*, (Downers Grove, Illinois: Intervarsity Press, 1993).

3   Marsden, pp. 371-372.

4   Carl L. Becker, *The Heavenly City of the Eighteenth-Century Philosophers*, (New Haven: Yale University Press, 1932), pp. 14-15,32.

5   Johnson, *Darwin On Trial*, p. 116.

6   Francis Crick, quoted by Phillip Johnson in *Wedge of Truth*, (Downers Grove,

Illinois: Intervarsity Press, 2000), p. 122.

7   Schaeffer, *Volume 5: How Should We then Live?*, p. 177.

8   Peter Singer, *Rethinking Life and Death – the Collapse of Our Traditional Ethics*, (New York: St. Martin's Griffin, 1994).

9   Ibid., pp. 187-222.

10   George Will, "Life and Death at Princeton," <u>Newsweek</u>, 13 September, 1999, p80.

11   Gene Edward Veith Jr., *Postmodern Times: A Christian Guide to Contemporary Thought and Culture*, (Wheaton, Illinois: Crossway Books, 1994), p. 50.

12   David Barton, p. 285.

13   Alexis de Tocqueville, Democracy in America: Specially Edited and Abridged for the Modern Reader, Richard D. Heffner, editor (New York: Penguin Books, 18984).

14   Ibid, p. 282.

15   Ibid. pp. 280-281.

CHAPTER FOURTEEN

A LAND AT WAR WITH ITSELF

A house divided against itself cannot stand.
Abraham Lincoln (1809-1865)

September 11th, 2001, thrust Americans headlong into the center of the complex world of international terrorism. Burned indelibly into our souls, that fateful day will forever haunt our dreams. We all felt the same horror and stunned disbelief as planes sliced the mirrored face of the World Trade Center, bursting into torrents of fire. We were hypnotized by unthinkable images, transfixed by the smoke tumbling steadily into a clear autumn sky. Revulsion crept into our bones as the towers collapsed into heaps of shattered glass, broken concrete, and twisted steel. An enemy unlike any previously known had pierced the heart of our homeland.

In the days that followed, a unity not seen since Pearl Harbor swept the country. Americans bound together with the pride of freedom remembered. Senators and Representatives stood side by side on the steps of our nation's capitol singing *God Bless America*. Cities around the world hushed for a moment of silence in recognition of our tragedy. In that grievous moment, there were no Democrats; there were no Republicans. We were Americans— and proud of it.

Three days later we shared our National Day of Prayer and Remembrance with the world. Images of soot-covered firefighters, fatigued policemen, and haggard citizens captured our thoughts. Heroes struggled day and night to rescue whomever they could—many losing their own lives trying to save others. Too often, these rescuers found only the broken bodies of the dead. We listened to heart-felt eulogies and eloquent prayers. Billy Graham's weathered face and unsteady gait betrayed both his age and his battle with Parkinson's disease, but his words rang with clarity, power, and truth for the world to hear. Though new to office and doubted by many, President George W. Bush rose with compassion, humility, and resolve to comfort a grieving nation at its moment of crisis. With broken voice and gracious words, he called Americans to recognize the best of who we are.

> The days of national unity, thought, and reflection slid into the darkening shadows of distant memory. Within a few short years, America lay deeply divided as if cleaved by a brutal medieval battle-ax.

The Lord's Prayer then arose from the still of that great cathedral, the lyrics echoing through the ancient halls of mortality with peaceful haunting. Light streamed through the great stained glass windows drawing our spirits heavenward. As the last strain faded into silence, bittersweet grief hung in the air. Each was captured by the solitude of her heart. Each examined his soul for what was supreme, grasping for meaning. Tears washed away the trivialities of life; only the treasured remained. In that moment America was beautiful.

A Fading Memory

However, those days of national unity, thought, and reflection slid into the darkened shadows of distant memory. Within a few short years, America lay deeply divided as if cleaved by a brutal medieval battle-ax. We all heard the agonized screams of victims soon to burn alive. We all witnessed the horrific images of men and women leaping to their deaths to escape the resulting inferno. As we surveyed the vacant lower Manhattan skyline, grief and disbelief welled within and sorrow hung heavy in our souls. But how we processed the events that followed evidenced two diametrically opposed underlying worldviews. Looking back on that painful day Americans gaze through two distinctly different lenses.

Three years later the world watched our country unabashedly disembowel itself during the 2004 presidential campaign (Bush vs. Kerry). Bitter partisan invective divided the nation. America's unified commitment to fight the war on terror collapsed as national debate degenerated into little more than political mudslinging. Losing sight of the enemy, we turned our guns upon ourselves and freely conceded a key principle of victory. In *The Art of War* Sun-tzu counsels, "If they are united, cause them to be separated."[1] A strategic victory al-Qaeda could never gain on their own was given to them for nothing.

As President Bush strove to defend the American people from a second attack, criticism against him betrayed a profound underlying division in our country. The animosity we witnessed may have even emboldened those seeking our destruction, making a tremendously difficult task yet more difficult. Undoubtedly, those who wished our ruin watched with perverted glee. With each passing news cycle, a wedge was driven ever deeper into America's soul. The voices of the far Left grew bolder, showing greater contempt for our President than for the nineteen terrorists who leveled the Twin Towers, claiming nearly 3,000 innocent American lives—than for Abu Mussab al-Zarqawi who brutally beheaded his captives as the world watched in horror.

The world listened to accusations from the floors of Congress, angry cries from the halls of free press, and impassioned speeches from political leadership. On October 16, 2003 Senator Kennedy relentlessly assailed the President from the Senate floor, "Before the war, week after week after week after week, we were told lie after lie after lie after lie."[2] On February 8, 2004 former vice president Al Gore shouted to a roaring crowd, "He betrayed this country! He played on our fears!"[3] Allegations the President concocted the war prior to 9/11 for political gain, that he targeted civilians in Afghanistan, and that he knowingly lied to America and misled the world to gain access to Iraqi oil flew fast and furious. Hollywood colluded with obscenities and films fueling anti-American sentiment on a global scale.

It is no surprise that international opinion slowly turned against us. A skeptical world only needed to believe the words of our own senior statesmen, the relentless pulsation of our own media, and the Hollywood elite. The terrorists undoubtedly drew strength from this reckless invective, gaining perverse pleasure and twisted satisfaction as they watched Americans turn upon themselves like a pack of rabid wolves.

But where did this division come from? With the war effort under a continuous and withering assault, America nearly left Iraq before securing victory. Polls repeatedly revealed Americans wanted the troops home more than they wanted to win the war. A Rasmussen survey in revealed 49% of respondents wanted to bring the troops home, only 42% believed we should win the war first.[4] Here we must answer the painful question of why.

> The terrorists undoubtedly drew strength from this reckless invective, gaining perverse pleasure and twisted satisfaction as they watched Americans turn upon themselves like a pack of rabid wolves.

Even though the traditional struggle for political power is forcefully in play, the animosity inside Washington finds deeper roots. Its true strength lies not in core partisan ideology but, once again, in the greater battle of worldviews. To make moral distinctions, there must be a standard by which all things are judged. Whether at the personal, national, or international level, a moral compass must exist to differentiate good from evil. Recall Jean-Paul Sartre's assertion, *no finite point has meaning unless it has an infinite point of reference.*[5] The fundamental dilemma facing America today is the lack of agreement on who determines this infinite point of reference, if one even exists at all.

Postmodern thought refutes the existence of such an infinite point of reference. "Truth" is what is true for you; "truth" is what is true for me. There is no Universal Truth against which all else is measured. However, this formulation stands justice on its head. The defenders (America) of the once universally recognized "good and right" now become the despised aggressors. This leaves the United States impotent, unable to stand against tyranny. The unwitting acceptance of this worldview sets the table for massive social upheaval. The unfortunate events surrounding Abu Ghraib reflected this sad reality.

The Devastation of Moral Equivalency

The coverage of Abu Ghraib demonstrated with stunning clarity the growing unwillingness of many in the national media to differentiate between the noble efforts of the American military and the tyranny of Saddam's brutal regime. When the Abu Ghraib story broke, night after night Americans, and the entire world, underwent a prolonged visual assault of what transpired in that Iraqi prison in graphic detail. For thirty-two consecutive days the New York Times ran front-page stories expounding the abuses.[6] Senior politicians repeatedly denigrated American troops in front of the international community. *Had they forgotten world opinion never forms in a vacuum?*

On May 10th, 2004, with coverage of the Abu Ghraib scandal at a fevered pitch, Senator Edward Kennedy noted on the senate floor, "President Bush asked, 'Who would prefer that Saddam's torture chambers still be open?' Shamefully, we now learn that Saddam's torture chambers reopened under new management: U.S. management." As grievous as the Abu Ghraib scandal was, far more regrettable was the fact seasoned politicians did not distinguish between the Ba'ath Party's longstanding institutional use of torture to retain political power and the greater mission of the United States military to end that cruelty.

In contrast to the daily barrage depicting American disgrace at Abu Ghraib, the abuses of Saddam Hussein, many of which occurred in that very prison, were not broadcast in parallel to help explain what compelled the American presence in Iraq to begin with. Our media possessed video footage of Saddam's regime gruesomely cutting off fingers, amputating hands, hacking out tongues while guards chant Saddam's praises, cutting off ears with razor blades, walking blindfolded men off the tops of buildings, mercilessly beating helpless people tied to posts, and worse. Instead of broadcasting these images the media chose to display photos devastating to our national pride over and over again, permanently etching those images into our minds.

Reflecting on the media's unwillingness to report the enemy's brutality during the Abu Ghraib scandal, Nick Shultz wrote "Seeing, and Believing: The torture tapes the media are ignoring" for the *National Review Online* on June 17, 2004:

> Earlier this month, National Review Online obtained a
> four-minute video of Saddam-era torture at the Abu Ghraib
> prison in Iraq. Many of us here who discussed the matter
> are ourselves unable to watch the whole video. Some could
> not get beyond the furious, ecstatic chanting of torturers as

they raised swords, celebrating their own dementia in the depths of a man-made hell. What to do with the video was a matter of debate here. On principle this is newsworthy— and weighing heavily on our deliberations was the fact that a group of United States senators held a press conference on June 2 [2004] during which they showed the horrific video and near no one covered it.... Some Westerners, including some who did not support the war in Iraq, frankly may not understand the evil that was the Saddam Hussein regime. You watch—or try to—the four-minute video and you *see* the unbearable evil that was—and that is no more because of the sacrifice of American and Coalition blood.[7]

Around the world the words "Abu Ghraib" instantly evoked images of menacing German Shepherds or naked men stacked in human pyramids. Through the deliberately graphic, repeated, and sensational coverage by the American media, this story needlessly became an international symbol of American shame. Rather than reflecting the heroism of the voluntary American soldier willing to lay down his or her life to secure another's freedom, the *New York Times* and other mainstream media outlets made certain that America, and the world at large, repeatedly saw our sons and daughters as pornographic, power hungry sadists.

> Rather than reflecting the heroism of the voluntary American soldier willing to lay down his or her life to secure another's freedom, the mainstream media made certain that America, and the world at large, repeatedly saw our sons and daughters as pornographic, power hungry sadists.

While Abu Ghraib dominated the headlines, a parallel story demonstrated American compassion and grace. It could have been widely publicized, but was not. After the 1991 war Saddam imprisoned seven Iraqi businessmen at Abu Ghraib for allegedly using American dollars. After serving their time each had his right hand amputated and his forehead tattooed permanently marking him as a criminal. The world never heard these Iraqi men received prosthetic hands under the care of a plastic surgeon in Houston, free of charge. Afterward, one of the Iraqi men, Salah Zinad, expressed his gratitude. This "gave us new hope for life... This hand will remind us of the fine and wonderful people here [Americans]... We have been able to open the big prison—the prison of Iraq."[8]

As the war progressed America seldom heard the heartfelt appreciation of many Iraqis. This letter from an Iraqi mayor should have been headline news from New York to Los Angeles but remained in obscurity:

> To the Courageous Men and Women of the 3d Armored Cavalry Regiment, who have changed the city of Tall' Afar from a ghost town, in which terrorists spread death and destruction, to a secure city flourishing with life.
>
> To the lion-hearts who liberated our city from the grasp of terrorists who were beheading men, women and children in the streets for many months.
>
> To those who spread smiles on the faces of our children, and gave us restored hope, through their personal sacrifice and brave fighting, and gave new life to the city after hopelessness darkened our days, and stole our confidence in our ability to reestablish our city....
>
> I have met many soldiers of the 3d Armored Cavalry Regiment; they are not only courageous men and women, but avenging angels sent by The God Himself to fight the evil of terrorism.
>
> The leaders of this Regiment; COL McMaster, COL Armstrong, LTC Hickey, LTC Gibson, and LTC Reilly embody courage, strength, vision and wisdom. Officers and soldiers alike bristle with the confidence and character of knights in a bygone era. The mission they have accomplished, by means of a unique military operation, stands among the finest military feats to date in Operation Iraqi Freedom, and truly deserves to be studied in military science. This military operation was clean, with little collateral damage, despite the ferocity of the enemy. With the skill and precision of surgeons they dealt with the terrorist cancers in the city without causing unnecessary damage.

God bless this brave Regiment; God bless the families who dedicated these brave men and women. From the bottom of our hearts we thank the families. They have given us something we will never forget. To the families of those who have given their holy blood for our land, we all bow to you in reverence and to the souls of your loved ones. Their sacrifice was not in vain. They are not dead, but alive, and their souls hovering around us every second of every minute. They will never be forgotten for giving their precious lives. They have sacrificed that which is most valuable. We see them in the smile of every child, and in every flower growing in this land. Let America, their families, and the world be proud of their sacrifice for humanity and life.

Finally, no matter how much I write or speak about this brave Regiment, I haven't the words to describe the courage of its officers and soldiers. I pray to God to grant happiness and health to these legendary heroes and their brave families.

NAJIM ABDULLAH ABID AL-JIBOURI
Mayor of Tall 'Afar, Ninewa, Iraq[9]

Why is this mayor's assessment of American soldiers so different from some politicians in Washington? On December 4, 2005, only two months before the letter of thanks written by the Iraqi mayor, John Kerry noted during an interview with Bob Schieffer on *Face the Nation*, "And there is no reason, Bob, that young American soldiers need to be going into the homes of Iraqis in the dead of night, terrorizing kids and children, you know, women…"[10] Addressing our efforts in Afghanistan, then Senator Obama shared similar sentiments on August 13, 2007, "We've got to get the job done there and that requires us to have enough troops so that we're not just air-raiding villages and killing civilians."[11]

Here we see two diametrically opposed views of the U.S. military effort taking shape. One demonized the American soldier, not recognizing the valor and moral authority with which he or she fought. The other saw courage beyond belief. One dominated the press; the other held at bay. The mainstream media and some of our senior political leaders failed to help Americans, and the world, comprehend the nature of freedom's enemy.

Why did the press obfuscate the clear moral distinction between American GI's and Saddam's brutal regime? Why were the hundreds of stories evidencing America's goodwill kept from the headlines day after day? Why did the *New York Times* choose instead to run fifty-three front-page stories about *American abuses* at Abu Ghraib? It was not to expose some great cover-up. The military began its investigation of this serious lapse of professionalism and supervision prior to the story going public.

The answer lies in the devastating conviction of moral equivalency. Recall the primary tenet of postmodernism—there is no Universal Truth. "Truth" is what is true for you; "truth" is what is true for me. All sides stand on level ground. The only perspective banned from a postmodern world is one that claims to know the Right. The unforgivable sin? To impose that view on others through military force. To the postmodern mind, this marks the epitome of narrow-minded arrogance. Here we find the source of the Left's anti-military passion. And when this passion explodes, it rends our nation in two.

During the State of the Union Address on January 9, 2002, President Bush used the phrase "Axis of Evil" to specifically identify the countries of Iraq, Iran, and North Korea. In doing so he implicitly claimed to know the good. Gaining the endorsement of Congress, President Bush then led the coalition of the willing to forcibly remove Saddam from power. It is difficult to imagine anything more offensive to a postmodern mind. America, under the leadership of President Bush, had committed the unforgivable sin.

As punishment, the postmodern media denigrated the American effort and President Bush at every turn while turning a blind eye to the evils under Saddam. This was their way of shouting to the world, "America really doesn't claim to know the Right. Bush claims to. But the rest of us don't!" Saddam's men starved babies in view of mothers, gouged out the eyes of children as terror stricken parents watched in horror, and repeatedly raped wives and daughters as husbands and fathers agonized helplessly. They slowly immersed innocent victims in vats of acid and used electric drills to bore holes into the hands and fingers of prisoners. But these stories were held from public view. In their place we witnessed perhaps our single greatest shortcoming of the war (Abu Ghraib) over and over and over again. In this manner a press appeased their guilt-laden, postmodern souls

A second point follows closely after the first. If the press and postmodern politicians demonstrated America's lack of moral authority, it proved their initial position—the American led coalition had no right to invade Iraq. Even more, America had no right to "impose justice" through military force. Stripping America's moral authority around the world placed her on equal footing with Saddam's Iraq. Coverage of the war was no longer about America's struggle against terrorism; it was about which worldview would dominate American and world politics for the generation to come.

Regrettably, comparing the American soldier to Saddam's elite guard with "neutral objectivity" stripped our nation of its will to fight. Ours is a nation of ideals, a people who still deeply believe that truth and justice *are* the American way. *If we come to believe we are no different than those we oppose, if we no longer see ourselves as defenders of the good and the right, we lose our capacity to defend the freedoms we so dearly love.* The danger of being immersed in a culture of absolute moral neutrality is that we never fully grasp the horrors of despotism; we never really understand the wars we fight.

Neglecting another fundamental teaching of Sun-tzu places America in a most vulnerable position—we do not know our enemy.[12] We no longer recognize the face of evil. Do we remember the ovens of Dachau? The mass graves at Auschwitz? Too often we forget our place in world history—that wherever the voice of freedom rings, it rings in memory of the fallen American soldier. *But to understand these things, one must understand the nature of evil— the very capacity postmodern thought destroys.*

Why Georgia had to "Show Restraint" After the Russian Invasion

Postmodern thought litters the political landscape—though, at times, it is difficult to recognize. At first blush it often sounds sophisticated, intellectual, cool, and reasoned. Who could argue with such an evenhanded academic approach? "We must understand all sides without passing judgment."

However, because postmodern thought lacks certainty of the good, the right, and the true (it lacks Sartre's infinite point of reference), in the end, it strips America of the ability to defend liberty.

In August of 2008 Russia launched a massive invasion deep into the heart of Georgia. Once a former satellite state of the Soviet Union, Georgia stood as a fledgling, independent democracy. In fact, with the weight of Soviet oppression fresh in its memory, Georgia proudly sent troops to fight with the coalition of the willing to help secure freedom for the people of Iraq. Russia's invasion of this close U.S. ally posed a serious question to 2008 Presidential nominees Barack Obama and John McCain. How should the United States respond? The initial positions of the two candidates revealed stark contrast.

Senator McCain never trusted Vladimir Putin. After President George W. Bush notoriously noted he looked into Putin's eyes and gained a sense of trust, McCain quipped that when he looked into Putin's eyes he saw the letters "K.G.B." McCain immediately recognized the threat this invasion posed and supported a joint statement by Presidents of the former Soviet satellite states Poland, Estonia, Latvia, and Lithuania:

> We, the leaders of the former captive nations from Eastern Europe and current members of the European Union and NATO– Estonia, Latvia, Lithuania and Poland – are extremely concerned about the actions of the Russian Federation against Georgia. We strongly condemn the actions by the Russian military forces against the sovereign and independent country of Georgia.
>
> Following the unilateral military actions of the Russian military forces, we will use all means available to us as Presidents to ensure that aggression against a small country in Europe will not be passed over in silence or with meaningless statements equating the victims with the victimizers.[13]

Likewise, Senator Barrack Obama released a statement. However, he framed the invasion of a U.S. ally in an entirely different manner:

I strongly condemn the outbreak of violence in Georgia, and urge an immediate end to armed conflict. Now is the time for Georgia and Russia to show restraint, and to avoid an escalation to full scale war. Georgia's territorial integrity must be respected. All sides should enter into direct talks on behalf of stability in Georgia, and the United States, the United Nations Security Council, and the international community should fully support a peaceful resolution to this crisis.[14]

Note the differences between these positions. McCain strongly condemned the "actions by the Russian military" clearly placing guilt at the feet of Russia. Obama condemned only the "outbreak of violence." McCain adamantly refused to equate "the victims with the victimizers." Obama called for both "Georgia and Russia to show restraint."

Senator McCain immediately saw the Russian aggression for the evil it was and rose to confront our former cold war nemesis. Senator Obama viewed both Russia and Georgia with moral neutrality. Though Obama sounded intellectual, cool, and reasoned, in his immediate response he could not bring himself to directly condemn the Russian Bear. He only asked both sides to show restraint.

Some may argue Obama's status as a freshman Senator explains this hesitant reaction. However, two weeks later he made a statement revealing this was not the case. Reuters reported:

Democrat Barack Obama scolded Russia again on Wednesday for invading another country's sovereign territory while adding a new twist: the United States, he said, should set a better example on that front, too.

The Illinois senator's opposition to the Iraq war, which his comment clearly referenced, is well known. But this was the first time the Democratic presidential candidate has made a comparison between the U.S. invasion of Iraq and Russia's recent military activity in Georgia.

"We've got to send a clear message to Russia and unify

our allies," Obama told a crowd of supporters in Virginia. "They can't charge into other countries. Of course it helps if we are leading by example on that point."[15]

This statement is remarkable. While campaigning to become President of the United States, Barack Obama publicly claimed Russia's unilateral invasion of a fledgling democracy was morally equivalent to the action of America (and the other 47 countries in the coalition of the willing) in Iraq.

America and her allies moved against Saddam as a last resort, and only after six months of build-up and negotiations with a clear expression of intent. Not only was Saddam one of the cruelest dictators of modern times, he had twice invaded neighboring states and was responsible for the deaths of some two million people. That Senator Obama considered these events morally equivalent can only be explained by postmodern thought.

Because postmodern thought cannot claim to know the Right, it looks to the surrounding culture as a guide. Three days after Russia's invasion of Georgia, in a more considered and extended statement Barack Obama appealed to the world body for help. "We should continue to push for a United Nations Security Council Resolution calling for an immediate end to the violence."[16] However, Obama did not appreciate that Russia was one of five nations holding veto power on the very council to which he appealed.

> *The purposeful lack of distinction between ourselves and those who seek our destruction divides the American public in the War on Terror—and this lack of moral clarity shall prove our undoing.*

The Death of Good and Evil

The purposeful lack of distinction between ourselves and those who seek our destruction divides the American public in the War on Terror—and this lack of moral clarity shall prove our undoing. As reviewed above, the mainstream media and some of our political leadership consistently portray America in a poor a light while suppressing stories of American heroism and the brutality of foreign despots.

We see this same phenomenon of sweeping moral equivalency at work in the United Nations. The inability to discern good from evil has rendered this institution impotent, unable to discriminate between the oppressor and the oppressed. All nations are given equal footing.

For example, the United Nations Human Rights Commission investigates human rights violations in countries around the world. In May of 2001 the United States was voted off the commission. Sudan was subsequently appointed and Libya given the chair. An amazing aspect of this story was that Sudan was in the midst of one of the largest acts of genocide in modern history. Over the previous seventeen years, the Sudanese government witnessed two million of its people killed and four million more displaced, largely to gain access to oil fields.[17]

We witnessed this again on September 23, 2008 when President Bush and Iranian President Mahmoud Ahmadinejad, shared the same stage, addressing the United Nations as equals. How can this be? According to the Anti-Defamation League, over the years Ahmadinejad repeatedly called for Israel's destruction:

> Today, it is clear that Israel is the most hated regime in the world... It is not useful for its masters [the West] anymore. They are in doubt now. They wonder whether to continue spending money on this regime or not...But whether they want it or not, with God's grace, this regime will be annihilated and Palestinians and other regional nations will be rid of its bad omen. (March 11, 2010)

> The Zionist regime wants to establish its base upon the ruins of the civilizations of the region...The uniform shout of the Iranian nation is forever 'Death to Israel.' (October 10, 2009)

> The Zionist regime (Israel) is going towards its final collapse after 60 years of aggression. The final solution would be a referendum on Palestine's future... (September 18, 2008)

> With God's help, the countdown button for the

destruction of the Zionist regime has been pushed by the hands of the children of Lebanon and Palestine... By God's will, we will witness the destruction of this regime in the near future. (June 3, 2007)

Israel is destined for destruction and will soon disappear. (November 13, 2006)

Israel must be wiped off the map. (October 26, 2005)[18]

Yet, the Iranian President is repeatedly invited to America to address the world with arrogant impunity. Tzipi Livni, Israel's Foreign Minister responded with anger, "Ahmadinejad's [United Nations] speech makes the situation absurd for an organization that raised the banner of 'Never Again' upon its establishment."[19]

The remarkable end of postmodern thought is that a nation who invades a developing democracy holds veto power in the world body intended to prevent this precise behavior. A man who calls for a second Holocaust speaks with impunity at the institution committed to never letting another Holocaust happen again. Yet, this is the reality of the postmodern world—it is the consequence of each voice being a voice unto itself, of Truth being no more than opinio.

Today the United States is on the same path that rendered the moral compass of the United Nations useless. In chasing the false god of autonomous freedom promised by postmodern thought, America is rapidly discarding her few remaining fixed points of reference. In the postmodern mind, every conceivable position is considered equally valid. This not only explains our nation's lack of unity in the War on Terror, it explains why some politicians turn either to Europe or to the United Nations for moral clarity. It is better to submit to the moral judgment of a world body than to commit the sin of claiming to know Truth ourselves.

This explains why some politicians turn either to Europe or to the United Nations for moral clarity. It is better to submit to the moral judgment of a world body than commit the sin of claiming to know Truth ourselves.

As the reader will see, our Founding Fathers' Judeo-

Christian worldview provided the ability to discern good from evil—an ability essential to the preservation of liberty. This worldview provided the moral basis for America's *Declaration of Independence* and the rule of law. Thomas Jefferson once queried, "And can the liberties of a nation be thought secure if we have lost the only firm basis, a conviction in the minds of the people that these liberties are the gift from God?"[20,21]

Without the concept of higher Truth, the ability to differentiate between good and evil is lost. In the United Nations each nation is given moral equivalence to the next. Under postmodern thought one idea carries no more weight than another. Each man's "truth" becomes a voice unto its own, a mere personal preference tossed on a tumultuous sea of competing ideas. Without the concept of fixed Truth, we become a land at war with itself.

Notes

1   Sun-tzu, *The Art of War*, (United States of America: Barnes & Noble Books, 1994), p. 168.

2   Ted Kennedy, Senate Floor Remarks, Thursday, 16 October, 2003.

3   Al Gore, Tennessee Democratic Rally, February 8, 2004.

4   Rasmussen Reports "49% Say Bring Home the Troops, 42% Say Win the War First," August 8, 2008.

5   Francis Schaeffer, *The Complete Works of Francis Schaeffer Volume 1: He is There and Not Silent*, (Westchester, Illinois: Crossway Books, 1988), pp. 277-278.

6   New York Times Streak of Page One Stories on Abu Ghraib ends at 32 Days! (UPDATED: 34 of 37 Days) www.freerepublic.com/focus/f-news/1145998/posts

7   Nick Shultz, "Seeing, and Believing: The torture tapes the media are ignoring", *National Review Online*, 17 June, 2004.

8   Jennifer Lehner, *The Washington Times*, "Seven Iraqi victims view 'Remembering Saddam'", May 27, 2004.

9   Mayor Najm Abdullah Abid Al-Jijouri. http://powerlineblog.com/archives/013133.php#013133, Feb 13, 2006.

10   John Kerry, Interview with Bob Schieffer, Face the Nation (CBS News), Sunday, December 4, 2005.

11   Barack Obama, "Obama: U.S. Troops in Afghanistan Must Do More Then Kill Civilians," Fox News, August 14, 2007, http://www.foxnews.com/story/0,2933,293187,00.html

12   Sun-tzu, p. 215.

13   Joint Statement on Russia's aggression in Georgia by the Presidents of Poland, Estonia, Latvia & Lithuania, "Equating the Victims With the Victimizers," August

9, 2008, www.johnmccain.com

14   Statement from Barack Obama on the Grave Situation in Georgia, August 8, 2008, www.barackobama.com

15   Barack Obama, "Obama: Russia, U.S. should not 'charge into' other countries" *Tales from the Trail*. Reuters Blogs, August 21, 2008. http://blogs.reuters.com/ trail08/2008/08/21/obama-russia-us-should-not-charge-into-other-countries/

16   Barack Obama, "Obama's Statement on Georgia," Real Clear Politics, August 11, 2008, http://www.realclearpolitics.com/articles/2008/08/obamas_statement_on_ georgia.html

17   United States Holocaust Memorial Museum, www.ushmm.org/conscience/index. utp?content=sudan/sudan.php, 20 November, 2004.

18   Anti-Defamation League, http://www.adl.org/main_International_Affairs/ ahmadinejad_words.htm?Multi_page_sections=sHeading_2

19   Tzipi Livni, "Livni: Ahmadinejad speech makes mockery of UN vow of 'never again,'" Barak Ravid, Haaretz Correspondent and News Agencies, September 24, 2008.

20   Thomas Jefferson, *Notes on the State of Virginia*, (Philadelphia: Matthew Carey, 1794), Query XVIII, p. 237.

21   David Barton, *Original Intent: The Courts, the Constitution, & Religion*, (Aledo, Texas: Wallbuilder Press, 2003), p. 46.

CHAPTER FIFTEEN

AMERICA'S POSTMODERN COURTS

*I do not believe that the meaning of the Constitution was forever "fixed"
at the Philadelphia Convention.... Nor do I find the wisdom, foresight
and sense of justice exhibited by the framers particularly profound.*
Supreme Court Justice Thurgood Marshall (1908-1993)

That all societies will be governed is a fact indelibly written on the pages
of human history. In the absence of higher moral principle, those who
make decisions make them because they can—because they have power. As
the rule of law breaks down, Samuel Rutherford's Lex Rex (Law is King)
becomes Rex Lex (The King is Law). Those in power gain autonomous
freedom and the common man is left without appeal. This is the story of
socialist rule.

On June 23, 2005, alarms rang across the country but few recognized
what had just transpired. Following *Kelo v. New London*, local governments
could seize private property for strip malls, condominiums, and yacht
clubs—all with the Supreme Court's blessing. Private citizens suddenly faced
the threat of eviction from their homes and businesses. For the first time in
American history, local governments could transfer prime real estate from
one private citizen to another for the sole reason of increasing tax revenue.
The unthinkable was now settled law.

How did this happen? How could the Supreme Court revoke the historic civil right of the private ownership of property? The answer lies in the inevitable erosion of law in a postmodern world—a world without a fixed point of reference. The chaos of such a world is unimaginable.

The World of the Autonomous Court

Once we understand the power of a postmodern worldview, *Kelo v. New London* begins to make sense. The hallmark of postmodern philosophy is the absence of any fixed point of reference. The concept of a transcendent "Truth" vanishes into the Byzantine past; everything is subject to personal preference. Words no longer mean what they once did. "Public use" becomes "public benefit."

In a postmodern world, even the founding documents of the United States are open to individual interpretation. One opinion holds no more weight than another. Though our Founding Fathers never intended this to happen, a mere five American citizens—five Supreme Court Justices—now hold the keys for titanic social change. *Absent a fixed understanding of the Constitution, a postmodern Supreme Court is free to wander wherever it will.*

Nothing portrays this battle over the meaning and authority of the Constitution more clearly than the highly unusual opening of the 112th Congress. On January 6, 2011—*for the first time in United States history*—Congressional leaders read the U.S. Constitution on the floor of the House of Representatives.

In 2010, Republicans achieved the greatest electoral comeback since 1938. Driven by the massive impact of the Tea Party movement the newly elected Republican majority wanted to symbolize their renewed pledge to the principles of limited government, fiscal responsibility, and Constitutional fidelity. By reading the Constitution, Republican leadership signaled a desire to return to the fixed principles of our nation's founding. This defines one side of the debate.

Ezra Klein, a staff writer for the *Washington Post*, expressed the opposing view with uncanny clarity when asked about the reading of the Constitution. In an interview on MSNBC Klein noted:

Q: [MSNBC's Norah O'Donnell] You heard all the different politicians talking about the Constitution. Well, this is what's going to happen. When Republicans take over next week, they're going to do something that apparently has never been done in the 221-year history of the House of Representatives. They are going to read the Constitution aloud. Is this a gimmick?

A: [Ezra Klein] Yes, it's a gimmick. [laughs] I mean, you can say two things about it. One is that it has no binding power on anything. And two, the issue of the Constitution is not that people don't read the text and think they're following. The issue of the Constitution is that the text is confusing because it was written more than 100 years ago and what people believe it says differs from person to person.[1]

Note the last sentence, "The issue of the Constitution is that the text is confusing... and what people believe it says differs from person to person." Rephrasing Klein only slightly almost defines postmodern thought: "The meaning of the Constitution is what people believe it is and its meaning differs from person to person."

Destroying the concept of a fixed Constitution by saying its meaning varies from person to person creates a serious problem. *Once the rule of law is freed from the Constitution's original intent, on what basis should judges judge? What standard provides the basis for law?* The empathy of those seeking their version of social justice? The personal perspectives of five Supreme Court Justices? The interest of the collective good? The financial interests of the State? Shadows of socialism lie beyond the doorway of a "living, breathing, Constitution."

> *Once the rule of law is freed from the Constitution's original intent, on what basis should judges judge? What standard provides the basis for law?*

Government compassion sounds so noble when first introduced. "We want every American to have access to healthcare." These words resonate with every good and patriotic citizen, yet, for Barbara Wagner, they ended with the elite deciding what medical care she could and could not receive. What holds true of healthcare holds true of law. To preserve our liberty, *we the people* must have something higher than the good will of government to which we can appeal.

Just as Plato and Hippocrates defined the two poles of thought for medicine, we find two poles of thought for the rule of law. Like Hippocrates, one pole submits to a "fixed Truth" preserving liberty for the common man. Like Plato, the other pole claims *autonomous freedom* leaving the elite with power to act as they see fit—here, the elite define the rights and privileges of the common man.

Defining the Poles

A painting by Paul Robert beautifully portrays the traditional worldview of men such as Samuel Rutherford and Sir William Blackstone. Painted in 1905, *Justice Lifts the Nations* is a massive work of art hung in the stairwell of the old Supreme Court building in Lausanne, Switzerland. Judges passed by it when going to hear a case. The painting questions, "How shall the judges judge? How shall they rule so law is not arbitrary?"

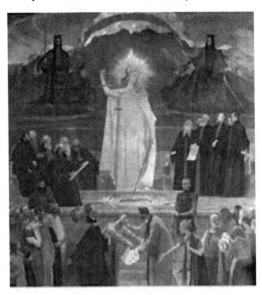

In the foreground, people wait for their case to be heard. Behind them stand the judges, looking toward the center of the picture at Justice. Robert portrays Justice as a woman robed in white with flowing golden hair. Lacking the blindfold she so commonly wears, Justice stands with eyes wide open. Her right hand holds the golden scales of justice; her left grasps the sword of

Truth. The sword points downward to a book lying open before her as she instructs the judges. On the book appear the words, "*LA LOI DE DIEU*" which means "The Law of God." Here, a fixed moral code provides the foundation for both law and justice. The rights of man are secure.

This painting stands in stark contrast to a lecture given eight years earlier at Boston University Law School. In 1879 the famed and brilliant legal scholar, Oliver Wendell Holmes Jr., outlined a second position in his speech, *The Path of Law*. As a confirmed Darwinist,[2] Holmes rejected the possibility of a higher law to which he was subject. In the naturalistic worldview God is excluded by definition—this makes an appeal to "The Law of God" irrational. Left without higher moral law, just as Peter Singer did for medicine, Holmes was free to create a new basis for law. He begins by separating law from morality:

> I wish, if I can, to lay down some first principles for the study of this body of dogma or systematized prediction which we call the law... I wish to point out an ideal which as yet our law has not attained.
>
> The first thing for a businesslike understanding of the matter is to understand its limits, and therefore I think it desirable at once to point out and dispel a confusion between morality and law...[3]

Holmes recognized a link between law and a society's moral life; "The law is the witness and external deposit of our moral life. Its history is the history of the moral development of the race."[4] But, reminiscent of Plato, Holmes lacks a fixed source of knowledge for what "moral" is. Commenting on this lecture, former Supreme Court clerk and retired Berkeley law professor Phillip Johnson states,

> This lecture has been so influential in shaping the thinking of American lawyers that it might be described as almost part of the Constitution. Holmes urged his audience of future lawyers to put aside all notions of morality and approach

law as a science, basically the science of state coercion. The reason people ask lawyers for advice, said Holmes, is not because they want to hear about morality but because they want to escape the unpleasant consequences that the law will inflict on them if they violate some rule. Therefore, [quoting Holmes] "if you want to know the law and nothing else, you must look at it as a bad man, who cares only for the material consequences which such knowledge [of the law] enables him to predict, not as a good one, who finds his reasons for conduct, whether inside or outside of it, in the vaguer sanctions of conscience."[5]

For Holmes, morality does not inform law but law defines morality. Right does not dictate what is legal; rather, what is legal determines what is right. As law evolves, so does morality. This is the antithesis of the painting by Paul Robert. These two men (Robert and Holmes) portray the difference between post-Reformation and postmodern law. The first provided an anchor to secure the common man's freedom. The second freed the elite to rule with autonomy.

The fact that America is a constitutional republic protects us from totalitarianism and gives us reason for hope. As a democracy, power returns to the people every two years in the form of elections. But as a constitutional republic, those elected to positions of authority live under the rule of law set forth in our nation's constitution; thus, the power of our elected representatives is limited and not arbitrary. These two principles secure the rights of *we the people* against the abusive power of government.

However, as Kelo v. New London so vividly illustrates, Americans can still lose their liberty—Americans can elect postmodern politicians who do not respect the principle of a fixed Constitution and the rule of law.

Why Postmodern Law is Inherently Unstable

In his book *Postmodern Times*, Gene Edward Veith discusses the link between postmodern thought and totalitarianism at some length. First he describes the ideology of a postmodern society, contrasting it to that of the modern age being left behind:

> Modernists believe in determinacy; postmodernists
> believe in indeterminacy. Whereas modernism emphasizes
> purpose and design, postmodernism emphasizes play and
> chance. Modernism establishes a hierarchy; postmodernism
> cultivates anarchy. Modernism values the type; postmod-
> ernism values the mutant. Modernism seeks the *logos*, the
> underlying meaning of the universe expressed in language.
> Postmodernism, on the other hand, embraces silence....
>
> Postmodernism attempts to re-order thought and culture
> on a completely different basis, accepting reality as a social
> construction... What kind of edifice can be built on such a
> foundation, or rather on the rejection of all foundations?[6]

Both the modernist and the postmodernist are naturalists in that they believe humanity is the end result of a random, purposeless process. However, where the modernist seeks to find order through science, the postmodernist revels in chaos. The more intellectually incongruent something is, the more awe it inspires. Aristotelian logic and Reason are useless against the truly postmodern thinker. "Truth" is what is true for me.

A foundation that rejects all foundations is inherently unstable. Freedom finally attained complete autonomy but only for a moment. Why? This worldview has one overwhelming shortcoming—when there is disagreement, who arbitrates? To what higher law can one appeal? Consensus will not last forever. Eventually someone will dispute another's freedom, demanding limits. Unlimited freedom that does not impose on another can only be found on a deserted island inhabited by one person. The moment a second arrives, conflict will ensue. What then? Who has the final word? *Whoever holds power.* If not restrained by higher law society will be governed by Nietzsche's übermensch.

The absence of a transcendent moral authority creates a colossal power

The absence of a transcendent moral authority creates a colossal power vacuum. When society no longer submits to the "laws of nature" and the "laws of God," power arbitrates—and power is arbitrary.

vacuum. When society no longer submits to the "laws of nature" and the "laws of God," power arbitrates—and power is arbitrary. Arbitrary power is precisely the bondage from which our Founding Fathers struggled so tirelessly to free themselves. Without a higher moral authority *Lex Rex* (Law is king) becomes *Rex Lex* (King is law). The new king is whoever wields power. When this happens, the common man loses his ability to hold the government to a fixed higher moral law. He falls subject to the whims of those in power and no longer is free. "Societal law" reigns supreme. History witnessed this during the Middle Ages with an autonomous church. History witnessed this yet again during the last century in the gulags, concentration camps, and killing fields. In every case, death was the result, not freedom.

When America moved into late modernity, higher education set aside its Christian consensus and replaced the "laws of nature" and "the laws of God" with "the laws of science." At this stage in our nation's development, we removed our *infinite point of reference*, but we still thought in terms of thesis and antithesis. Americans, even the intellectually elite, still believed in "right" and "wrong," only the standard against which they were measured had changed. Rather than viewing "right" and "wrong" in moral terms, these concepts were defined by what could be proven by science. This led to the rise of the social sciences. If a given social position could be "proven" superior, it became "right."

But ultimately, who determines this "societal law?" Sociologists? Bioethicists in the ivory towers of Princeton? Judges? The Supreme Court? Veith phrases it this way:

> Moreover, excluding transcendent values places societies beyond the constraint of moral limits. Society is not subject to the moral law; it makes the moral law. If there are no absolutes, the society can presumably construct any values that it pleases and is itself subject to none. All such issues are only matters of power. Without moral absolutes, power becomes arbitrary. Since there is no basis for moral persuasion or rational argument, the side with the most power will win. Government becomes nothing more than the sheer exercise of unlimited power, restrained neither by law nor by reason…

To be sure, most postmodernists today do not explicitly advocate totalitarianism. On the contrary, they intend their positions to be liberating, freeing oppressed groups from the "one truth" proclaimed by oppressive cultural forces. And yet it is difficult to see how their premises could in any way support a free society. Clearly, democracy rests on the *opposite* of postmodern tenets—on the freedom and dignity of the individual, on humane values, on the validity of reason, on God rather than the state as the source of all values, on a transcendent moral law that constrains both the tyranny of the state and the tyranny of individual passions.[7]

As American culture sets aside the "laws of nature and of nature's God," a power vacuum is created, one our judicial system is more than willing to fill. As judges embrace postmodern thought, the rule of law itself is gradually set aside. The very concept of our Constitution providing a fixed point of reference is antithetical to the postmodern mind. "Right" and "wrong" become personal preferences because the words "right" and "wrong" now mean "what is right or wrong at the moment for myself." To impose a universal definition of "right" and "wrong" is simply intolerable. *Thus, judges who no longer recognize the Constitution's original intent—including the limited role of the judicial system—become the greatest and most direct threat to our liberty.*

Even as history can be rewritten when it becomes no more than a "language game," so can law. Does "public benefit" really mean "public use?" Or is this just another language game used by the Court to transfer power to the elite?

Washington, We Have a Problem. Do You Copy?

Between October 27, 1787, and May 28, 1788, Alexander Hamilton, James Madison, and John Jay wrote a series of 85 articles known as the *Federalist Papers*. Hamilton was an influential delegate at the Constitutional Convention, Madison became our fourth President, and Jay served as the first Chief Justice of the Supreme Court. Why should we think these men understood the Constitution's original intent? Because they helped create it, they were eyewitnesses to the debates that took place.

Hamilton, Madison, and Jay published the *Federalist Papers* to educate the public about the proposed Constitution and gather support for its ratification. As such, these articles comprise one of the most authoritative sources available when discerning the intent of the framers. To understand the foundations of our country we must understand the writings of these men. The fact that our nation's framers created the longest ongoing constitutional republic in the world attests to the wisdom and power of their ideas.

Alexander Hamilton specifically addressed the balance of power with respect to the courts in the *Federalist Paper*, Number 78:

> Whoever attentively considers the different departments of power must perceive, that, in a government in which they are separated from each other, **the judiciary, from the nature of its frustration, will always be the least dangerous to the political rights of the constitution; because it will be least in a capacity to annoy or injure them.** The Executive not only dispenses the honors, but holds the sword of the community. The legislature not only commands the purse, but prescribes the rules by which the duties and rights of every citizen are to be regulated. **The judiciary, on the contrary, has no influence over either the sword or the purse; no direction either of the strength or of the wealth of the society; and can take no active resolution whatever. It may truly be said to have neither FORCE nor WILL, but merely judgment**; and must ultimately depend upon the aid of the executive arm even for the efficacy of its judgments.
>
> This simple view of the matter suggests several important consequences. **It proves incontestably, that the judiciary is beyond comparison, the weakest of the three departments of power**; that it can never attack with success either of the other two; and that all possible care is requisite to enable it to defend itself against their attacks. **It equally proves, that**

though individual oppression may now and then proceed from the courts of justice, the general liberty of the people can never be endangered from that quarter; I mean so long as the judiciary remains truly distinct from both the legislature and executive. For I agree, that "there is no liberty, if the power of judging be not separated from the legislative and executive powers." And it proves, in the last place, that as liberty can have nothing to fear from the judiciary alone...[8] (Bold emphasis added. Capitalized "FORCE" and "WILL" were in the text.)

Examining the original intent of those who crafted our Constitution shows how far our country has drifted from its fixed point of reference. According to Hamilton in the *Federalist Papers,* "The judiciary... has no influence over either the sword or the purse... and can take no active resolution whatever. It may truly be said to have neither FORCE nor WILL, but merely judgment." These are remarkable words considering the state of affairs today. In his book, *Restraining Judicial Activism,* David Barton briefly outlines the problem:[9]

In *Compassion in Dying v. Washington* and in *Quill v. Vacco,* courts reversed the results of elections in Washington and New York in which the citizens had voted to forbid physician-assisted suicides;

In *Missouri v. Jenkins,* although citizens voted down a proposed tax-increase, the courts nevertheless ordered the tax to be levied;

In *Yniguez v. Arizona,* the courts reversed the results of the vote by Arizona citizens that English be the official language of the State;

In *LULAC v. Wilson* and *Gregorio T. v. Wilson,* the courts suspended the results of the California vote to withhold

State-funded taxpayer services from those who are *illegally* in the country;

In *Carver v. Nixon*, the courts set aside the results of a statewide election wherein Missouri citizens voted to approve campaign financing reform by setting limits on candidate contributions from individuals;

In *U. S. Term Limits v. Thornton* and *Thorsted v. Munro*, the courts overturned the results of elections in which citizens in Arkansas and Washington had voted to limit the terms of their elected officials; and

In *Romer v. Evans*, the courts overturned a constitutional amendment approved by Colorado citizens to forbid awarding special, rather than just equal, rights to homosexuals.

The Massachusetts Supreme Court Dictates Law

One of most brazen acts of unconstitutional judicial activism was when the Massachusetts Supreme Court mandated the state Congress pass legislation legalizing same sex marriages in November 2003. This stood the separation of powers on its head. Congress is to make law; the judicial branch is to apply that law to the courts. Here, four justices forced the creation of law against the will of the Congress. Four of seven judges set social policy for the state. *The Founding Father never intended Judges to mandate social policy. In fact they expressly denied them this power.* Quoting Hamilton, the judiciary is to have "neither FORCE nor WILL, but merely judgment." How far we have come from the original intent our Founding Fathers!

In his book *Men in Black*, Constitutional scholar Mark Levin discusses the events surrounding this case in some detail.[10] By a vote of four to three, the Massachusetts Supreme Court determined that denying homosexual marriages violated the Massachusetts Constitution. To rectify this problem, they altered the legal definition of marriage to mean "the voluntary union of two persons as spouses to the exclusion of all others."[11] In doing this the Massachusetts Supreme Court appealed to the Ontario Court of Appeal in Canada to legitimize this ruling, not the U. S. or Massachusetts Constitutions! But more was yet to come.

After altering the definition of marriage, the court notified the Massachusetts legislature that it had 180 days to pass a law legalizing gay marriage. The legislature responded with legalizing "civil unions" that would confer all rights of marriage to gay couples except one—the title of marriage. The court's reply? Legalizing "civil unions" was insufficient; legalizing "gay marriages" was mandated, forcing the legislature to pass a law legalizing gay *marriage*.

Levin follows this discussion with these words:

> Despite this opinion, the Massachusetts legislature was not deterred. It went ahead with a constitutional convention. It passed the civil union law and an amendment to the state constitution banning same-sex marriage, but the earliest it will appear on the ballot for ratification is 2006.
>
> Nevertheless, shortly after midnight on May 17, 2004— the end of the court's deadline to institute gay marriage— municipal clerks began handing out marriage licenses to same-sex couples in Massachusetts. As the Associated Press reported, "As of Monday, Massachusetts joins the Netherlands, Belgium, and Canada's three most populous provinces as the only places worldwide where gays can marry."[12]
>
> Four of seven justices of the Supreme Judicial Court of Massachusetts—with a stroke of a pen—abolished hundreds of years of tradition and law over the strong objections of the legislature. And as these activist justices undoubtedly intended, their ruling will have consequences well beyond their jurisdiction and Massachusetts borders.[13]

Same Sex Marriage in California

A similar situation in California provided another clear example of a subculture of judges that no longer submit to the rule of law. On March 7, 2000 Californians passed Proposition 22 by a margin of 61.4% to 38%. This largely replicated 1977 law clearly defining marriage as the union of one man and one woman.

During February 2004, San Francisco Mayor Gavin Newsom gave a directive that same-sex marriage licenses could be issued; over the next nine days, 3,175 such licenses were obtained. Even though Proposition 22 explicitly defines marriage as the union of a man and a woman, Judge Ronald Evans Quidachay of the San Francisco Superior Court openly defied California State law by allowing the licenses to stand.[14] The fact that the Judge Quidachay ruling was overturned as a flagrant violation of California State law does not make it any less remarkable. He demonstrated a judge can openly defy the very law he swore to uphold without repercussion.

On May 15, 2008 an unelected elite* overturned the will of the people. By a vote of 4-3, the California Supreme Court declared Proposition 22 unconstitutional. Once again the people of California were forced to express their will, this time by amending the California State Constitution with Proposition 8. Once again the measure passed; once again the Left sued to overturn the will of the people in court.

In pursuit of social change, voices on the far Left cheer court rulings that overturn the will of the people. Yet, each time the far Left moves toward *autonomous freedom* through judicial fiat, *we the people* lose another piece of liberty. As Susette Kelo learned, a court with enough power to change the definition of marriage is a court with enough power to seize your home. Using the courts in a way the Founding Fathers never intended unleashes an unstoppable force that, in the end, will consume our freedom.

---

* In California, the Governor appoints new Supreme Court Justices. To remain on the Court, the new Justice must then be "retained" during the next general election. However, should the electorate vote to remove a sitting Justice, the Governor then appoints another new Justice. This means while voters can remove a Justice, they do not actually elect the members of the Supreme Court.

The Courts Seize Control of Citizenship

Mark Levin's exceptionally well-researched book, *Men in Black*, provides over 200 pages of documentation and analysis of how the U.S. Supreme Court gradually usurped power that it was never intended to have. *Men in Black* should be read by every thoughtful citizen in America, liberal and conservative alike.

Levin begins chapter seven by citing Article I, Section 8 of the Constitution: "The Congress shall have power to… establish an uniform rule of naturalization."[15] He notes that through the action of the courts, the status of both legal and illegal aliens is:

> …increasingly indistinguishable from that of citizens. So while the Constitution gives to Congress the sole authority to determine how many immigrants may enter the country, how many immigrants can become citizens of the United States, and whether those immigrants should be able to avail themselves of the benefits of U.S. citizenship, the Court has chosen on several occasions to ignore the express direction of the founders and usurp that authority for itself.[16]

To defend that assertion Levin cites several examples. In the 1971 case of *Graham v. Richardson,* the Supreme Court decided that Arizona did not have the right to establish minimum length of state residency requirements before an alien began receiving welfare benefits.[17] In the 1973 case of *In Re Griffiths,* the Supreme Court found a state could not deny non-citizens the right to take the bar exam and become licensed, practicing attorneys.[18] In the 1976 case of *Hampton v. Mow Sun Wong,* the Supreme Court ruled that the government could not make citizenship a requirement for civil service jobs such as the Post Office, the Health, Education, and Welfare Departments or other federal agencies.[19] In the 1977 case of *Nyquist v. Mauclet,* the Supreme Court found it was unconstitutional for New York to require aliens to apply for citizenship before receiving financial aid for education. In the 1982 case of *Plyler v. Doe,* the Supreme Court extended the term "person" in the Fourteenth Amendment to illegal aliens. It compelled Texas to provide free

THE BATTLE FOR AMERICA'S SOUL

public education to children of illegal immigrants.

These decisions are often defended by arguing that the Court provides relief for the unfortunate when the legislature fails to do so. "The Court is creating freedom and finding equality for oppressed people. Isn't that what the United States stands for? 'Give me your tired, your poor, your huddled masses yearning to breathe free...'"

Recognizing many illegal aliens come to the United States to find a better life, many Americans are sympathetic to their plight. Yet, however compassionate we feel regarding immigration policy, the judiciary is clearly usurping authority the Founding Fathers never intended it to have. Setting the Constitution aside threatens the rule of law, especially when the courts assume a legislative posture. Recall Hamilton's warning, "For I agree, that 'there is no liberty, if the power of judging be not separated from the legislative and executive powers'."

Whether dealing with property rights, immigrant rights, or the definition of marriage, postmodern thought frees the Court from the Constitution's original intent. In doing so, it transfers power from *we the people* to government. For this reason, an autonomous judiciary marks the single gravest threat to American liberty because it leaves the common man without appeal. *What is law, is right.* Only shadows separate this from Marcus de Sade's formulation: *what is, is right.*

Sorting Out the Justices

Four days after *Kelo v. New London* the Supreme Court offered a second ruling revealing the worldviews of the individual Justices. *McCreary County v. ACLU of Kentucky* addressed the constitutionality of displaying the Ten Commandments in a county courthouse. In a 5-4 ruling, the Supreme Court ruled in favor of the ACLU finding the presence of the Ten Commandments unconstitutional. The revealing detail lies in how the individual Justices voted.

Four of the five Justices voting in favor of local governments seizing private property in *Kelo v. New London*, voted against displaying the Ten Commandments in *McCreary County v. ACLU of Kentucky*. These were the Leftward leaning Justices Ruth Bader Ginsberg, John Paul Stevens, David

Souter, and Stephen Breyer.

Three of the four Justices voting against local governments to seize private property in *Kelo v. New London*, voted in favor of displaying the Ten Commandments in *McCreary County v. ACLU of Kentucky*. These were the Rightward leaning Justices William Rehnquist, Antonin Scalia, and Clarence Thomas.

The correlation is illuminating. Those Justices who found it constitutional to display the Ten Commandments were unwilling to change the intent of the Fifth Amendment—their worldview retained the concept of a fixed moral code. These Justices recognized the Supreme Court's freedom was not autonomous, acknowledging a fixed moral code is the basis for the rule of law; this is represented by the Ten Commandments.

Those Justices who found it unconstitutional to display the Ten Commandments declared the Fifth Amendment words "public use" really meant "public benefit"—their worldview rejected the concept of a fixed code of any sort, Biblical or Constitutional. The foundation of these Justices' worldview rested on the principle of *autonomous freedom*. Released from the constraints of the Constitution's original intent, they determined it constitutional for the government to seize a private home and give it to a developer for State interests. This is socialism pure and simple, a governing philosophy antithetical to individual liberty.

Our postmodern press and socially elite declare the Judeo-Christian worldview irrational and dangerous. Yet, which worldview is most dangerous to the soul of America? The evidence speaks for itself. Logic explains the reason why socialist states throughout history expelled religion. A government constrained by the "laws of nature and nature's God" must recognize its citizens have "certain unalienable rights." If a socialist government wishes complete autonomy, it must free itself of this restraint. If "religion" remains in the public square, it must be a religion devoid of absolutes. Its teachings can only be "helpful suggestions."

The Future of Freedom

Archimedes once said, "Give me a lever long enough and a fulcrum on which to place it, and I shall move the world." Where our courts act as the lever, public education serves as the fulcrum—and the two work in concert to alter the very fabric of the American way of life. When a postmodern Supreme Court set aside legal precedent and the original intent of the Constitution, it began to tinker with society to effect social change. One of the primary targets was public education.

Notes

1   Ezra Klein, Norah O'Donnell, MSNBC Daily Rundown, December 30, 2010.

2   Phillip Johnson, *Reason in the Balance*, (Downers Grove, Illinois: Intervarsity Press, 1995), p 143.

3   Oliver Wendell Holmes, Jr., *The Path of Law*, 1897.

4   Ibid.

5   Phillip Johnson, p. 140.

6   Veith, *Postmodern Times*, p. 33-34.

7   Ibid., pp. 159-160.

8   Alexander Hamilton, *The Federalist*, pp. 490-491.

9   David Barton, *Restraining Judicial Activism*, (Aledo, Texas: Wallbuilder Press, 2003), p. 8.

10   Levin, pp. 83-85.

11   Goodridge v. Dept. of Pub. Health, 440 Mass. 343 (Mass. 2003).

12   Ken Maguire, "Marriage-liscence applications given to same-sex couples in Massachusetts." Associated Press, May 7 2004.

13   Mark Levin, pp. 84-85.

14   Dean Murphy, *New York Times*, "San Francisco Judge Rules Gay Marriages Can Continue," 20 February, 2004.

15   The Constitution of the United States, Article I, Section8., June 21, 1788.

16   Levin, p. 107.

17   Ibid., p. 107.

18   Ibid. p. 113.

19   Ibid., p. 108.

CHAPTER SIXTEEN

FIGHTING FOR OUR FUTURE

The future of a nation lies in the minds of its youth.

They waited, magnificent and shimmering in the moonlight as a cool breeze caressed their steel-grey hulls. Shadows crept across the harbor's rippled surface. In the distance, the soft lapping of water gradually replaced the sounds of music. Anticipating the warmth of the morning sun, ironwood trees peered through the night. With unending gaze, they watched the liquid silver of light dance atop gentle waves pushed up by occasional boats ferrying men through the dark. For the first time in five months the battleships all lay at anchor, secure in their proper places. General Short grouped his planes tightly together on the open airstrips to protect them against possible sabotage. Pearl Harbor slept unaware that fire would soon devour her core naval strength and ravage her air defenses. When America awoke hours later, 1,100 men on board the USS Arizona lay imprisoned in a watery grave. Many of her finest were dead.

December 7, 1941, galvanized Americans, arming them with the strength, courage, and resolve needed to fight and win a prolonged and brutal war. The next four years witnessed 291,557 Americans killed and another 670,846 wounded. Yet, in spite of severe setbacks and overwhelming casualties, America refused to consider defeat. America's "Greatest Generation" rose to answer the call of history. These heroes secured their place on the world's stage as defenders of freedom. They fought with moral clarity under the noble banner of liberty. When Japan surrendered and Hitler's armies finally laid down their arms, our nation's shores were secure once again. Americans of every political stripe could live at peace in the greatest country the world has known.

With this privilege comes responsibility—the responsibility to preserve the precious freedom purchased with American blood. Simply living in this land of liberty does not guarantee this inheritance. America must retain both the ability to see where danger lies and the willingness to confront it. Hidden from view, the battle for America's soul threatens this capacity in future generations. Because this struggle remains largely unrecognized, Americans are rapidly losing the war for the hearts and minds of their own children. If stripped of the ability to make moral judgments, these young Americans will prove impotent should history call on them once again to defend their land of liberty.

> The absence of moral touchstones ends with complete disregard for authority. In our postmodern world, many of America's youth now agree with Jean-Paul Sartre: we live in an absurd universe where meaning is found in self actualization, though no one action is better or worse than another.

American culture is changing. Just a few years ago moral discretion was an assumed part of society. Parents could communicate precisely with a simple phrase such as "Be good" or "Do what you know is right." In a postmodern world, the words "good" and "right" ring hollow, stripped of significance. As assuredly as night follows day, the steady diet of naturalism in our public schools has created a culture without boundaries. Time plus chance plus Darwinian selection pressure leaves no rational basis for a transcendent meaning of life.

The absence of moral touchstones ends with complete disregard for authority. In our postmodern world, many of America's youth now agree with Jean-Paul Sartre: we live in an absurd universe where meaning is found in self actualization, though no one action is better or worse than another. Ours is becoming an age of non-Reason. The ability to see the American experiment as a great and noble cause, as the last great beacon of hope for the oppressed, is rapidly disappearing.

Those seeking to rework the fabric of American life know that if they could change *how children think* it would only be a matter of time until society followed. *For the future of a nation lies in the minds of its youth—and this is where the courts began.*

How Five Supreme Court Decisions Forever Changed Education

1) In 1947, the Supreme Court ruling of *Everson v. Board of Education* forever altered the face of American education. It ruled: "The First Amendment has erected a wall between church and state. That wall must be kept high and impregnable. We could not approve the slightest breach."

In reaching this decision the Supreme Court appealed to a letter Thomas Jefferson wrote to the Danbury Baptists on January 1, 1802. Paradoxically, as an anti-federalist, Jefferson wrote this letter to assure the Danbury Baptists the federal government would never restrict their freedom of religion. In the context of this letter, Jefferson's "wall" was intended to protect religion against the imposition of government, not government against the potential influence of religion. *Everson v. Board of Education* assigned to Jefferson's words a meaning precisely the opposite of his intent.

If Jefferson thought the influence of religion on government to be so perilous, why would he say:

> And can the liberties of a nation be thought secure if we [lose] the only firm basis, a conviction in the minds of the people that these liberties are the gift of God?[1,2]

2) The following year, 1948, in *McCollum v. Board of Education* the Supreme Court moved even more aggressively against religious teaching in schools. Even with parental consent, elective religious classes paid for by the church were declared unconstitutional. Justice Felix Frankfurter declared:

> Separation means separation, not something less.... It is the Court's duty to enforce this principle in its full integrity.... Illinois has here authorized the comingling of sectarian with secular instruction in the public schools.

The Constitution of the United States forbids this.[3]

Compare Justice Frankfurter's statement to Article III of the Northwest Ordinance. The Northwest Ordinance outlines the requirements for statehood for prospective territories. It passed the House on July 21, the Senate on August 4, and was signed by President Washington on August 7, 1789. Article III states:

> Religion, morality, and knowledge, being necessary to good government and the happiness of mankind, school and the means of education shall forever be encouraged.[4]

The year the Northwest Ordinance passed into law, 1789, is significant—this was the year James Madison submitted the Bill of Rights to Congress. The same men who mandated that "Religion, morality, and knowledge, being necessary to good government and the happiness of mankind, school and the means of education shall forever be encouraged," were the same men who declared that "Congress shall make no law respecting an establishment of religion, or prohibiting the free exercise thereof" in the First Amendment. Clearly, these men saw no conflict between the First Amendment and teaching religion in public schools.

Just as clearly, Justice Frankfurter ignored the original intent of Congress when they passed the Bill of Rights. His words, "The Constitution of the United States forbids this," express blatant disregard not only for the Founding Fathers' original intent, but also for the Constitution itself.

3) On June 25th, 1962, the Supreme Court made another astonishing break from tradition. For the first time in U.S. history,[5] a decision was given *citing no legal precedent* when *Engel vs. Vitale* struck down school prayer. This stands in marked contrast to the 1892 Supreme Court ruling in *Church of the Holy Trinity vs. the United States*. Here, the Supreme Court provided *87 citations* defending the ruling: "No purpose of action against religion can be imputed to any legislation, State or national, because this is a religious people... this is a Christian nation."[6]

4) The following year, 1963, *again without legal precedent*, the Supreme Court ruled in *School District of Abington Township vs. Schempp* that Bible reading and Bible teaching in public schools was unconstitutional.[7] This was remarkable because biblical material had been a part of formal public education for over 300 years. The very framers of the Constitution had gone through Christian based education. Higher education itself began as a vehicle to teach Christian principles.

5) In 1980 the Supreme Court ruled the posting of the Ten Commandments in public schools unconstitutional. *Stone vs. Graham* read in part, "If the posted copies of the Ten Commandments are to have any effect at all, it will be to induce the schoolchildren to read, meditate on, perhaps to venerate and obey, the Commandments." It concluded. "This... is not a permissible state objective..."[8]

In August 2003 the process came full circle with a tragic touch of irony. Federal Judge Myron Thompson ordered Alabama Supreme Court Chief Justice Roy Moore to remove the Ten Commandments from the public area of the State Judicial Building. Beginning with *Everson v. Board of Education* the Supreme Court removed God from education. Now, having received this Godless education, a federal judge removed God from the Court. The irony? Judge Myron Thompson was born in 1947, the year the Supreme Court ruled on *Everson v. Board of Education*. Following in the footsteps of Nietzsche, the only world that Judge Thompson knew was a world in which God was dead.

But what has come to pass as a byproduct of this achievement?

Culture's Destiny Foreshadowed in the Minds of Youth

Having stripped God from public education, large portions of the past three generations reject the concept of a fixed Truth. Allan Bloom described this phenomenon a quarter of a century ago. In 1987 he began his book, *The Closing of the American Mind*, with this reflection:

There is one thing a professor can be absolutely certain
of: almost every student entering the university believes,

or says he believes, that truth is relative. If this belief is put to the test, one can count on the students' reaction: they will be uncomprehending. That anyone should regard the proposition as not self-evident astonishes them, as though he were calling into question 2 + 2 = 4.... The relatively of truth is not a theoretical insight but a moral postulate, the condition of a free society, or so they see it.[9]

The concept of Truth is seen as an outmoded thought form, a relic of the past. However, without Truth virtues such as honor, integrity, loyalty, honesty, discipline, and self-sacrifice vanish as their foundations are siphoned from society. Without Truth moral courage itself has no base on which to stand. If man is the measure of all things, self-restraint is a fading fiction, and altruism slips into the dustbin of forgotten history. Without Truth, heroism is dead. In its place we find manipulation of the masses.

> The concept of Truth is seen as an outmoded thought form, a relic of the past. However, without Truth virtues such as honor, integrity, loyalty, honesty, discipline, and self-sacrifice vanish as their foundations are siphoned from society.

The June 27, 1997, issue of *The Chronicle of Higher Education* contained two disconcerting examples that reflect current cultural trends in higher education. Unfortunately, these stories can be told hundreds of times over at nearly any university in the country.

In the first article, Kay Haugaard, a creative writing professor at Pasadena College, related a class discussion about Shirley Jackson's classic short story, "The Lottery." For the first time in her teaching experience, she encountered a class of students unable to morally condemn the practice of human sacrifice.

I was stunned: This [student] was the woman who wrote so passionately of saving the whales, of concern for the rain forests, of the rescue and tender care of a stray dog... For a moment I couldn't even respond. This woman actually couldn't seem to bring herself to say plainly that she was against human sacrifice...

I turned to Patricia, a 50-something, redheaded nurse.

She had always seemed an intelligent person of moderate views. "Well, I teach a course for our hospital personnel in multicultural understanding, and if it is part of a person's culture, we are taught not to judge, and if it has worked for them…"

At this point I gave up. No one in the whole class of more than 20 ostensibly intelligent individuals would go out on a limb and take a stand against human sacrifice…

The class finally ended. It was a warm night when I walked out to my car after class that evening, but I felt shivery, chilled to the bone.[10]

Robert Simon, who teaches philosophy and ethics at Hamilton College in upstate New York, wrote the second article. In discussing the basis for moral thought, he brought up the Holocaust for discussion.

"Of course I dislike the Nazis," one of my students commented, "but who is to say they are morally wrong?" Other students in my classes on moral and political philosophy have made similar remarks about apartheid, slavery, and ethnic cleansing. They make the assertion as though it were self-evident; no one, they say, has the right even to criticize the moral views of another group or culture.

Although groups denying the reality of the Holocaust have raised controversies on some college campuses, in more than 20 years of teaching college students, I have yet to meet even one student who has expressed doubts about whether the Holocaust actually happened. However, I have recently seen an increasing number of students who, although well-meaning, hold almost as troubling a view. They accept the reality of the Holocaust, but they believe themselves unable morally to condemn it, or indeed to make any moral judgments whatsoever.[11]

Within a decade of *The Closing of the American Mind's* publication, Bloom's thesis (that students now accept that Truth is relative) had reached its logical conclusion. College undergraduates once readily understood the absolute moral travesties of human sacrifice or genocide. But those days of moral clarity have faded. When Haugaard and Simon wrote these articles in 1997, many of today's lawyers, doctors, and policy makers were students. God help us when America's political leaders and judges have lost all moral discernment as well.

A 22-year-old student taking these classes would have entered kindergarten the year the Supreme Court ruled (*Stone v. Graham*) that Kentucky's policy of posting the Ten Commandments in public classrooms was unconstitutional. Charles Carroll, signer of the *Declaration of Independence*, warned against such a ruling:

> [W]ithout morals a republic cannot subsist any length of time; they therefore who are decrying the Christian religion… are undermining the solid foundation of morals, the best security for the duration of free governments.[12]

With God expelled from America's public education, an alarming number of students graduating high school today cannot distinguish good from evil. Upon entering college they cannot say the Holocaust was morally wrong; they cannot categorically condemn human sacrifice. One may respond to this fact with a sense of shock, but it makes perfect sense; America's public education, media, and cultural elite preach postmodernism. *All fixed points of reference have been removed. What is right is what seems right at the moment.*

Enron's bankruptcy in late 2001 revealed one of the largest cases of corporate accounting fraud in American history. Enron employed some 22,000 people and claimed over $100 billion dollars in revenue during 2000. Kenneth Lay, it CEO, was found guilty on 10 of the 11 charges filed against him.

Less than seven years after the Enron scandal, the failure of Fannie Mae and Freddie Mac triggered the largest and most complex financial crisis since the Great Depression. Fannie Mae's CEO from 1999 to 2004, Franklin Raines, received approximately $90 million in compensation. Raines stepped down after the discovery of fraudulent accounting that overstated the earnings of Fannie Mae by over $6 billion. Approximately $50 million dollars of Raines compensation came in the form of bonuses based on these overstated earnings.

Is this unexpected? In November of 2008 the Josephson Institute released as survey of 29,760 students from 100 randomly selected high schools across the United States.

— 10% agreed with the statement: In sports, if you're not cheating, you're not trying hard enough.
— 23% admitted to stealing from parents or relatives.
— 36% admitted to cheating by copying an Internet document for a classroom assignment.
— 40% agreed with the statement: A person has to lie or cheat sometimes in order to succeed.
— 42% agreed with the statement: I sometimes lie to save money.
— 59% agreed with the statement: In the real world, successful people do what they have to do to win, even if others consider it cheating.
— 64% admitted to cheating on an exam.
— 77% believed they were better than most people when it came to doing what was right.
— 82% admitted to copying another student's homework.[13]

The Loss of Truth Ends with the Loss of Innocence

As all restraint is set aside, the loss of childhood innocence is staggering. In October 1999, the Public Broadcasting System (PBS) aired a documentary on "The Lost Children of Rockdale County." They investigated an outbreak of 200 cases of teenage syphilis. That was only the surface issue. What lay beneath? Writing for *City Journal*, Kay Hymowitz gave this description in her article "What's Wrong with the Kids?"

> The occasion for the show [The Lost Children of Rockdale County] was an outbreak of syphilis that ultimately led health officials to treat 200 teenagers. What was so remarkable was not that 200 teenagers in a large suburban area were having sex and had overlapping partners. It was the way they were having sex. This was teen sex as *Lord of the Flies* author William Golding might have imagined it, a heart-of-darkness tribal rite of such degradation that it makes a collegiate "hook up" look like splendor in the grass. Group sex was commonplace, as were 13-year-old participants. Kids would watch the Playboy cable TV channel and make a game of imitating everything they saw. They tried almost every permutation of sexual activity imaginable—vaginal, oral, anal, girl on girl, several boys with a single girl, or several girls with a boy... During some drunken parties, one girl might be "passed around" in a game. A number of kids had upward of 50 partners. Some kids engaged in what they called a "sandwich"—while a girl performs oral sex on one boy, she is penetrated vaginally by another boy and anally by yet another.[14]

Reading this is enough to make any parent physically ill. Thirteen years old! With this unbelievable level of sexual exposure, any concept of social restraint will be completely foreign to these children. And that was more than a decade ago. But there is more.

Simon Pulse, the children's literature division of publisher Simon & Schuster, published the "edgy" (positive descriptor) children's book *Rainbow Party* by Paul Riditis in 2005. The Crayola-colored, lipstick-laden cover looks innocent enough, but the subject matter is beyond many adults. The story begins with two girls in the shopping mall picking out multiple colors of lipstick for a "special party."

New to the scene of youth entertainment is the "rainbow party." Here girls perform oral sex on boys, while boys try to have as many colors applied to their genitalia as possible—giving the effect of a rainbow after multiple episodes of oral sex. This is not fiction: this is happening to children across America reaching down into elementary school.

Over half a century ago C. S. Lewis observed, "In a sort of ghastly simplicity we remove the organ and demand the function. We make men without chests and expect of them virtue and enterprise. We laugh at honor and are shocked to find traitors in our midst. We castrate and bid the geldings be fruitful."[15] We strip culture of all moral standards and teach our children they were "carelessly thrown up between two ice ages by the same forces that rust iron and ripen corn," yet are astonished by the resulting behavior. We incredulously ask with moral outrage, why the moral lapse at Abu Ghraib? But perhaps America should be thankful tragic events such as this are not repeated more often. Our culture cannot remove the foundations of morality, place our youth in the heat of battle, and then be shocked at a rare lapse of behavior—however devastating that lapse may be.

Will America realize there must be restraint if she is to survive? Has she reached the point of no return? If we destroy our youth, we destroy our future. Lacking a moral touchstone, Marquis de Sade prevails, "what is, is right."

> We stripped our children of all moral standards, yet are astonished by the resulting behavior... If we destroy our youth, we destroy our future.

Choosing which Road to Travel

America stands at the door of a new era, though not the wide-open door of autonomous freedom Nietzsche saw when he pronounced God dead. The door is behind us, about to close with latch drawn and bolt secured. We now stand in a room left only to ourselves, not being so bold as to declare God dead but deciding instead that He is obsolete. Like the sailors preceding Ulysses, we may have been seduced but this time by the Siren's song of *naturalistic materialism*. Our culture has no boundaries; we live in a world with no restraint. We sail on Nietzsche's sea without a shore, vainly searching the horizon to find a fixed point of reference. Anxiety mounts as night settles in.

America must see the thread woven through these examples. The traditional worldview of most Americans during WWII gave them the ability to persevere; they *knew* they were battling evil. A postmodern worldview cannot draw this conclusion because its philosophical premise is that the only evil is to make moral judgments. Postmodern students cannot condemn the Holocaust or state human sacrifice is morally wrong. Postmodern education strips children of their moral compass; 59% of students believe that, in the real world, successful people do what they have to do to win. Postmodern parents refuse to constrain their children's sexual behavior. Postmodern medicine ends with infanticide and active euthanasia. Postmodern law sacrifices private property on the altar of "public benefit."

In his book *Idols for Destruction*, Herbert Schlossberg reviews the concept of historicism, sometimes referred to as the "Doctrine of Inexorable Progress." This view states that as the history of mankind moves forward, change is progress and progress is good. Though often not consciously recognized, this view is widely held in American culture. Many believe that humanity moves along a line of continuous moral progress, always advancing.[16] Each new decision, each change of social mores, is viewed in isolation apart from the driving philosophy—unrecognized as a logical conclusion of the underlying worldview. This concept seduces the average American into accepting whatever is new. Each barrier of social restraint torn down by the ACLU, each time the Supreme Court rules counter to the original intent of the Founding Fathers, we move one step closer to *autonomous freedom*. To the far Left, this is "progress" by definition.

However, the "Doctrine of Inexorable Progress" is an illusion. In reviewing bioethical thought, this book reveals that America has not steadily advanced along a line; she has come full circle—returning once again to the troubled shores of ancient Greece. She finds herself at the same ethical crossroads faced by Plato and Hippocrates 2,500 years ago, contemplating State sponsored euthanasia and infanticide.

Before us lies a defining moment; America must decide which of two paths to follow. To the left lies the secular progressive movement where the pursuit of *autonomous freedom* eventually leads to the loss of individual liberty; the welfare of the State overwhelms the wellbeing of the individual citizen and our next generation cannot distinguish good from evil. To the right lies the worldview of our Founding Fathers where a higher moral code limits the State securing freedom for the common man.

American society now faces the real suggestion of redefining humans to be "fully human" on at four weeks of age. Some of the academically elite have proposed that we consider killing infants who do not "measure up." Not only are we destroying our children, we are contemplating infanticide. *My God, what have we become? Whose is this face in the mirror?* Society consumed individuality and the common man stands without appeal. For all of the progress postmodernism promised, we have succeeded only in returning to the shores of ancient Greece.

Our nation has at last come to the point of action. Having surveyed the dominant thought forms of western civilization, we find America stands at a divide in the road. As a nation *we the people* must choose one way or the other. Given these worldviews are diametrically opposed, to travel them both is impossible. An attempt to do so would rend our country in two; we would become a land at war against itself.

The Road of Ancient Rome

As the Age of Non-Reason dawns, what is to become of humanity? From Roman history, we learn that cultures do not survive when moral restraint is set aside. In Rome abuse of freedom led to the loss of moral standards, destruction of moral standards led to chaos, and chaos was exchanged for despotism. Despotism destroyed freedom, loss of true freedom led to apathy, apathy brought decay of culture, and decay of culture ended in death. The once great Roman Empire was no more. They had destroyed themselves from within. Schaeffer notes the parallels between the decline of Rome and the United States:

> Edward Gibbon (1737-1794) in his *Decline and Fall of the Roman Empire* (1776-1788) said that the following five attributes marked Rome at its end: first, a mounting love of show and luxury (that is, affluence); second, a widening gap between the very rich and the very poor... third, an obsession with sex; fourth freakishness in the arts, masquerading as originality, and enthusiasm pretending to be creativity; fifth, an increased desire to live off the state. It all sounds so familiar.[17]

279

We the people stand at a pivotal crossroads in American history—nothing less than the rule of law and the survival of culture as we have known it is at stake. Medicine must not forsake her Hippocratic roots and America must not forsake the faith of her Fathers, for the two are bound inextricably together. We must teach our children that life has more meaning than the vast emptiness naturalism mandates. Our Founding Fathers understood the necessity of a Judeo-Christian foundation for our nation. John Adams cautioned, "Our Constitution was made only for a moral and religious people. It is wholly inadequate to the government of any other."[18] George Washington similarly warned in his Farewell Address:

> And let us with caution indulge in the supposition that morality can be maintained without religion. Whatever may be conceded to the influence of refined education on the minds... reason and experience both forbid us to expect that national morality can prevail in exclusion of religious principle.[19]

United States District Judge Lawrence Karlton expressly set this wisdom aside on September 14th, 2005 when he ruled the words "under God" in the Pledge of Allegiance were unconstitutional. How could Judge Karlton believe he could interpret the Constitution's meaning more accurately than those who wrote it? The answer emerges under the light of *The Battle for America's Soul*. For the postmodern thinker, truth is what is true for me, history is what we choose to say it is, and the Constitution can be interpreted to further whatever political agenda is pressing at the moment. To the postmodern mind, Judeo-Christian restraint *is* the great evil of our day. Hence any evidence of God's authority over our nation must be swept from the public square.

This belief drives the ACLU's repeated suits to remove Christianity's symbols and influence wherever they are found. Following the model of Enlightenment thought, these lawsuits are presented as achieving "freedom from the tyranny of religion" by separating church and state. Certainly, one of the many privileges of living in the greatest country on earth is to passionately love America and not believe in God. However, Americans must recognize our nation's foundation, the rule of law, is rooted in the Judeo-Christian worldview. If this foundation is destroyed, another worldview will replace it. How is this accomplished?

In February of 2010 the North Carolina Department of Public Instruction laid out a piece of such a plan. The Department of Public Instruction proposed the high school United States history curriculum would eliminate material prior to 1877.[20] This curriculum modification conveniently eliminated the Founding Fathers, the Declaration of Independence, and the Constitution itself from the high school history curriculum. Removing these fixed points of reference opens the door to autonomous freedom.

However, the concept of attaining truly autonomous freedom is only a fiction, a fabrication of hopeful naïveté. That all mankind lives under law is the unavoidable fact of history. There are laws that enslave men's souls and there are laws that set men free. America must now choose what her foundation for law will be.

History is replete with examples of societies that set aside the intrinsic value of human life and a higher moral law to which all are subject, replacing it with the law of despotism. These societies often began with noble sounding causes but ended in destruction—the natural end of humanity when constraint is removed. In his Templeton Address "The Enduring Revolution," Charles Colson portrays this well:

> One writer called the modern age "the golden age of exoneration." When guilt is dismissed as the illusion of narrow minds, then no one is accountable, even to his own conscience.
>
> The irony is that this should come alive in this century, of all centuries, with all its gulags and death camps and killing fields. As G. K. Chesterton once said, the doctrine of original sin is the only philosophy empirically validated by the centuries of recorded history.
>
> It was a holocaust survivor who exposed the myth most eloquently. Yehiel Dinur was a witness during the trial of

Adolf Eichmann. Dinur entered the courtroom and stared at the man behind the bulletproof glass—the man who presided over the slaughter of millions. The courtroom hushed as a victim confronted a butcher.

Then suddenly Dinur began to sob, and collapsed on the floor. Not out of anger or bitterness. As he explained later in an interview what struck him at that instant was a terrifying realization. "I was afraid about myself," Dinur said. "I saw that I am capable to do this... Exactly as he."

The reporter interviewing Dinur understood precisely. "How was it possible for a man to act as Eichmann acted?" he asked. "Was he a monster? A madman? Or was he perhaps something even more terrifying... Was he normal?"

Yehiel Dinur, in a moment of chilling clarity, saw the skull beneath the skin. "Eichmann," he concluded, "is in all of us."[21]

Yehiel Dinur realized the potential of evil when a higher moral code is abandoned. Aleksandr Solzhenitsyn agreed when he received the 1983 Templeton Foundation Prize for Progress in Religion. Speaking of the Russian revolution he said, "[I]f I were asked today to formulate as concisely as possible the main cause of the ruinous Revolution that swallowed up some sixty million of our people, I could not put it more accurately than to repeat: '*Men have forgotten God; that's why all this has happened*'."

> *The postmodern world knows no bounds as the hands of time reshape the unthinkable into the thinkable.*

Two philosophies now battle for our hearts and minds and for the hearts and lives of our children. Each side yearns for freedom. The person of tradition yearns for the freedom that comes within a society ruled by law and higher moral code; the other yearns with Nietzsche for freedom from supreme law and higher moral code.

The attempt to redefine marriage, one of the most important social issues of our time, is one example. If marriage can be redefined by judicial fiat, why stop short at two men or two women? Why not three men? Or two sisters? Or one man and four women? Or a fathe and daughter or his under-aged son? Once "marriage" is open to revision there is no logical reason it must be limited to two people or why those two people cannot be related. *The postmodern world knows no bounds as the hands of time reshape the unthinkable into the thinkable.*

The postmodern media and far Left portray traditional values as "intolerant" and "judgmental," as the great evil of our time. However, every worldview, including postmodernism, makes judgments. Every individual has limits to what he or she will tolerate. Even the postmodern assertion "You can't judge other people" is itself a judgment.

Reversing Course

So, what can be done? Americans must first understand the relationship between worldviews and the chaos we find in the culture that surrounds us. The American public still recoils at the thoughts of infanticide and of local governments seizing private property. These two issues retain enough repulsion to awaken our citizens and politicians to the process ravaging our country. If our great nation is to survive, our classrooms and courtrooms must return to the foundations that created the greatest free county the world has known. America cannot afford to let another generation of her youth proceed through postmodern schools. To control education is to control the future of America.

In his remarkable book, *Why Johnny Can't Tell Right From Wrong,* William Kilpatrick relates the story of an eight-grade class being taught "values clarification." The teacher emphasized that students must determine what values were "right" for themselves; she explained outside influences were coercive manipulation. The class then selected its four most popular values: 1) Sex, 2) Drugs, 3) Drinking, and 4) Skipping school.[22] But the teacher had cut herself off at the knees. Once she taught a worldview based on complete autonomy, she no longer could provide moral guidance. Yet she had, she had guided them into a world of self-destruction. Her worldview imploded. Sadly, rather than an isolated incident this worldview dominates public education. *We the people* must understand the process that is eviscerating our country.

The hope of this great country lies with its people. Between New Jersey's ivory towers of Princeton University and California's Ninth Circuit Court of Appeals lies the heartland of America where the greatness of our country has not been forgotten, where the memory of our Judeo-Christian heritage lives on. Belief in the intrinsic value and dignity of every human—regardless of ethnicity—provides the moral clarity needed to sacrifice our sons and daughters for others. How often American soldiers place themselves in harm's way to save Iraqi and Afghan civilians will never be known. "Greater love has no one than this, that he lay down his life for another." Americans must not forget the historic source of this extraordinary honor and strength.

Americans have a heritage of courage and passion for freedom around the world. Though demagogued by those who seek *autonomous freedom*, the United States remains a beacon of hope and liberty to all who live under brutal oppression. However, our nation must recover its basis for human dignity and regain its fixed moral compass to continue to fight for the causes of justice. Is there hope? Yes, if Americans remember the foundations of freedom and recognize the postmodern politician when they enter the ballot box. For only with disciplined vigilance will America remain the greatest constitutional republic the world has ever known.

Notes

1   Tomas Jefferson, Notes to the State of Virginia, (Philadelphia: Matthew Carey, 1794). Querry XVIII, p. 237.

2   Barton, *Original Intent*, pp. 46.

3   McCullum v. Board of Education at 231, Frankfurter, J. (concurring).

4   *Constitutions* (1813), p. 364, "An Ordinance of the Territory of the United States Northwest of the River Ohio." Article III.

5   David Barton, "America's Godly Heritage," (Aledo, Texas: Wallbuilders, 1992), video presentation.

6   Barton, *Original Intent*, pp. 50, 155-160.

7   Ibid., pp. 160-165.

8   David Barton, *Original Intent*, pp. 170-172.

9   Allan Bloom, *The Closing of the American Mind*, (New York: Simon & Schuster, 1987), p. 25.

10   Kay Haugaard, "Suspending Moral Judgment: Students Who Refuse to Condemn the Unthinkable. A Result of Too much Tolerance?," *The Chronicle of Higher Education*, 27 June, 1997, Vol. XLIII, Number 42, pp. B4-B5.

11   Robert Simon, "The Paralysis of 'Absolutophobia'," *The Chronicle of Higher Education*, 27 June, 1997, Vol. XLIII, Number 42, pp. B5-B6.

12   David Barton, p. 168.

13   The Ethics of American Youth – 2008 Summary, Josephson Institute Center for Youth Ethics, November, 2008. http://charactercounts.org/programs/reportcard/index.html

14   Bernard Goldberg, *Arrogance: Rescuing America from the Media Elite*, (New York: Warner Books, 2003), pp. 241-242.

15   C. S. Lewis, *The Abolition of Man*, (New York: Simon & Schuster, 1996), p. 37.

16   Herbert Schlossberg, *Idols for Destruction*, (Nashville, Camden, Kansas City: Thomas Nelson Publishers, 1983), pp. 11-38.

17   Schaeffer, *Volume 5: How Should We Then Live?*. p. 227.

18   *The Works of John Adams—Second President of the United States*, (Boston:Little Brown, 1854), vol. IX, p.229.

19   George Washington, *Farewell Address*, 17 September, 1796.

20   Real History Reform: History Did Not Begin in 1877. http://realhistoryreform.org/

21   Charles Colson, "The Enduring Revolution: A Battle to Change the Human Heart", Templeton Address, University of Chicago, 2 September, 1993.

22   William Kilpatrick, *Why Johnny Can't Tell Right From Wrong*, (New York: Simon & Schuster, 1993), p. 81.

CHAPTER SEVENTEEN

THE IMPACT OF POSTMODERN POLITICS

If you look for truth, you may find comfort in the end;
If you look for comfort you will not get either comfort or truth
Only soft soap and wishful thinking to begin, and in the end, despair.

C. S. Lewis (1898-1963)

Without the concept of a fixed Truth, Americans find themselves living in a morally inverted universe. Good becomes evil and evil champions itself as the good. Columbia University clearly exemplifies this fact.

In September of 2007 Columbia University invited the Iranian president, Mahmoud Ahmadinejad. to speak on their campus. Driven by the postmodern ideal of "diversity of thought" Columbia gave one of the world's leading sponsors of terror a national platform here on American soil. Even more, Columbia University legitimized Ahmadinejad's call for Israel's destruction by granting it the respectability of academic debate. However, Columbia's effort to "listen to all sides evenhandedly" extends only so far.

During the unrest surrounding the Vietnam War, Columbia banned the Reserve Officer Training Corps (ROTC) from campus. In 2005, the faculty considered reversing this policy but once again refused the ROTC entry. In February 2011, a Columbia student, Anthony Maschek (an Iraq war veteran who sustained multiple gun shot wounds in Kirkuk), made another appeal to reverse this forty-year-old policy. With a sad sense of irony, the students who eagerly welcomed Mahmoud Ahmadinejad under the banner of "free speech" mocked the Purple Heart recipient with jeers, laughter, and catcalls when he spoke of his effort to secure true freedom for the citizens of Iraq.

The moral confusion that enables university students to applaud one of the world's leading sponsors of terror while deriding an American hero says nothing about freedom of speech. Instead, it speaks volumes about America's growing inability to distinguish between good and evil. History warns that the danger to a great society lies within; if left unchecked, the destruction of our moral compass will prove America's undoing.

Americans must understand the philosophical shift reshaping culture and American universities is reshaping the world of politics as well. As C. S. Lewis noted, "In a sort of ghastly simplicity we remove the organ and demand the function. We make men without chests and expect of them virtue and enterprise. We laugh at honor and are shocked to find traitors in our midst. We castrate and bid the geldings be fruitful."[1] Academia, the mainstream media, and the entertainment industry relish the autonomous freedom of postmodern thought. However, it is irrational to think political leaders can emerge from this culture and suddenly adopt a traditional worldview the moment they assume power. *The autonomous freedom championed in our universities steals both liberty and independence when it moves into politics.*

Because America remains a democracy, *we the people* still choose those who lead, set policy, make our laws, and appoint our judges and justices. Our Founding Fathers believed final power rested with the citizens, not with an entitled aristocracy. Only through complacency can this privilege of self-governance be lost. Every two years we go to the polls. It is here we must defend our freedom.

If the logical end of postmodern thought is the destruction of America's founding principles, how do voters recognize the postmodern politician? Not all Democratic leaders are postmodern, and not all Republicans hold a traditional worldview. In fact, most unwittingly blend these diametrically opposed worldviews at least to some degree. Political spin makes it difficult to separate one from the other. Rarely will one issue by itself reveal a politician's underlying philosophy. Politicians often base their positions on political expediency, not their personal worldview. However, trends can be revealing. Watch for these six tendencies to help detect postmodern thought in politics:

1) The disregard for the rule of law.
2) The transfer of power to government.
3) The appointment of postmodern Supreme Court Justices.
4) The appeal to foreign law.
5) The inability to move against reprehensible behavior abroad.
6) The acceptance of the concept of global governance.

* * *

1) Postmodern Politicians Disregard the Rule of Law

The end of Chapter Nine discussed Kierkegaard's belief that to have faith was to abandon Reason; to have faith was to believe in the absurd. Academia then pushed faith into the realm of non-reason. In doing so academia destroyed the "laws of nature and nature's God" as meaningful realities. With the landscape swept free of restraint, Chapter Ten witnessed the rise of Nietzsche's *overman* whose task was to overcome traditional limitations. *The truly postmodern thinker sees the rule of law as a matter of inconvenience, not as the fundamental principle that preserves our freedom.*

> The truly postmodern thinker sees the rule of law as a matter of inconvenience, not as the fundamental principle that preserves our freedom.

Michael Barone, author of *The Almanac of American Politics*, stands as one of the most brilliant political minds of our age. Published every two years since 1973, Barone's *Almanac* remains perhaps the most definitive analysis available for political trends in the United States. Barone's spontaneous mastery of obscure voting patterns is nothing short of encyclopedic. In brief, Michael Barone is not a newcomer to the political scene.

In March of 2009 Barone wrote an article for *The Washington Examiner* that should have brought the news cycle to a halt. His piece, "White House puts UAW ahead of property rights," detailed the events surrounding Chrysler's bankruptcy. Barone wrote:

Last Friday, the day after Chrysler filed for bankruptcy, I drove past the company's headquarters on Interstate 75 in Auburn Hills, Mich.

As I glanced at the pentagram logo I felt myself tearing up a little bit. Anyone who grew up in the Detroit area, as I did, can't help but be sad to see a once great company fail.

But my sadness turned to anger later when I heard what bankruptcy lawyer Tom Lauria said on a WJR talk show that morning. "One of my clients," Lauria told host Frank Beckmann, "was directly threatened by the White House and in essence compelled to withdraw its opposition to the deal under threat that the full force of the White House press corps would destroy its reputation if it continued to fight."

Lauria represented one of the bondholder firms, Perella Weinberg, which initially rejected the Obama deal that would give the bondholders about 33 cents on the dollar for their secured debts while giving the United Auto Workers retirees about 50 cents on the dollar for their unsecured debts.

This of course is a violation of one of the basic principles of bankruptcy law, which is that secured creditors — those who lended money only on the contractual promise that if the debt was unpaid they'd get specific property back — get paid off in full before unsecured creditors get anything....

The White House denied that it strong-armed Perella Weinberg. The firm issued a statement saying it decided to accept the settlement, but it pointedly did not deny that it had been threatened by the White House. Which is to say, the threat worked....

Think carefully about what's happening here. The White House, presumably car czar Steven Rattner and deputy Ron Bloom, is seeking to transfer the property of one group of people to another group that is politically favored. In the process, it is setting aside basic property rights in favor of rewarding the United Auto Workers for the support the union has given the Democratic Party....

Ordinarily you would expect these claims to be weighed and determined by the rule of law. But not apparently in this administration.

Obama's attitude toward the rule of law is apparent in the words he used to describe what he is looking for in a nominee to replace Justice David Souter. He wants "someone who understands justice is not just about some abstract legal theory," he said, but someone who has "empathy." In other words, judges should decide cases so that the right people win, not according to the rule of law.[2]

Barone concludes his piece with the observation, "We have just seen an episode of Gangster Government. It is likely to be part of a continuing series." Indeed, the way President Obama handled the bankruptcy of Chrysler marked a sad moment for America. He violated the rule of law in an open and explicit fashion and the nation rolled on without batting an eye.

2) Postmodern Politicians Transfer Power to Government

Chapter Eight noted that in the wake of Enlightenment thought, Voltaire's humanism could not bridge the gap between the common man and the rule of law. This was an impossible task given the elite's worldview. Having no basis for intrinsic human worth, Voltaire viewed the commoner with disdain, incapable of democracy and self-government. *The only rights the common man possessed were those graciously bestowed upon him by those in power. This is the philosophical basis of socialism—contempt for the common man.*

The stories of Barbara Wagner and Suzette Kelo reveal what this contempt means for the common citizen. Government compassion sounds so noble, but in the end, individual freedom is sacrificed on the altar of the "greater good." Nothing in modern times portrays this more clearly than the Patient Protection and Affordable Care Act (PPACA), otherwise known as Obamacare.

At the most basic level the PPACA shifts power from patients and physicians to Washington—and with this transfer of power comes the end of the historic patient/physician relationship. For centuries the implicit trust found in Hippocratic ideals characterized America medicine. In the days when the patient compensated the physician directly it was clear the physician served the patient. Physicians gladly devoted themselves to the wellbeing of the individual patient. Even if the patient was unable to pay, there was no confusion of where the physician's loyalties lay.

While universal healthcare does not make care free, it does consolidate power in one giant institution, the federal government.

However, government-controlled healthcare (as does non-catastrophic health insurance, only to a lesser degree) fundamentally changes this dynamic. Advocates of universal healthcare argue that medical care in Europe and Canada is "free." But in reality government run healthcare only shifts money from the free market to the taxpayer. Working citizens shoulder this cost either way. While universal healthcare does not make care free, it does consolidate power in one giant institution, the federal government.

Here lies the problem—whoever pays holds power. When Washington pays for American healthcare, the government gains power over medical decision-making. This impacts patients and physicians differently.

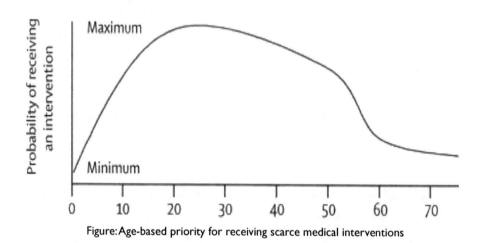

Figure: Age-based priority for receiving scarce medical interventions under the Complete Lives System

For patients, especially those on Medicare, the massive $14 trillion national debt weighs directly on the issue of access to care. In order to gain support for the PPACA, politicians pledged to cut $500 billion from

Medicare to "reduce the deficit." However, because expanding bureaucracies tend toward inefficiency rather that efficiency, finding $500 billion of actual savings is little more than wishful thinking. The alternative? Cut services. This is precisely what President Obama's healthcare advisor, Ezekiel Emanuel, outlined in his January 2009 paper. Recall Dr. Emanuel's graph explaining his Complete Lives System:

The difficulty of a single payer system for seniors is they have nowhere else to turn. Should the government follow Dr. Emanuel's advice and limit care for seniors, they will have no choice but to go without certain forms of healthcare. *Recall socialism's contempt for the common man. Here the contempt is directed toward seniors on Medicare.*

Physicians face a different threat altogether. Buried in the 2,700 pages of the Patient Protection and Affordable Care Act one finds 1,968 new or expanded governmental powers, 159 new federal agencies, and the transfer of unprecedented authority to the Secretary of Health and Human Services. For example, section 3007 details one of the nearly 2,000 new or expanded governmental powers. It reads, "The Secretary shall establish a payment modifier that provides for differential payment to a physician or a group of physicians... based upon the quality of care furnished compared to cost."[3] It then says the Secretary will define "the appropriate measures of cost."

After clearing away the legalistic verbiage, one finds the PPACA grants the Secretary of Health and Human Services the power to reduce physician reimbursement if an individual physician strays from what the Secretary considers "cost effective care." In other words, an unelected, unaccountable bureaucrat can bankrupt a physician who does not follow the federally mandated guidelines created by that same unelected, unaccountable bureaucrat.

Look at Dr. Emanuel's Complete Lives System once again. Under a universal healthcare system, the government gains the ability to set whatever standards it chooses. Under Section 3007 of the Patient Protection and Affordable Care Act, the government also gains the ability to force physicians to follow these guidelines (or to quit practicing medicine). This transfers enormous power to government. Physicians become tools of the State, and the days of Hippocratic medicine fade into forgotten history. Perhaps better than any other issue of our time, the PPACA displays the real world implication of postmodern politics.

3) Postmodern Politicians Appoint Postmodern Supreme Court Justices

When attempting to understand a politician's political philosophy, examine his or her attitude toward the Constitution and look at which Supreme Court Justices he or she admires. Taken together, these two closely related indicators reveal more about the underlying worldview than perhaps any other metric:

— Politicians holding a postmodern worldview believe in a "living, breathing Constitution" where its meaning changes with time. They look to Justices such as Ruth Bader Ginsberg and Stephen Breyer with satisfied approval. Appealing to the longstanding virtues of compassion and empathy, these individuals view the courts as agents of social progress by discovering new "liberties" in the law.

—Politicians holding a traditional worldview seek the Constitution's original intent. They turn with measured reassurance to Justices such as Clarence Thomas, Antonin Scalia, Samuel Alito, and John Roberts. These politicians believe the Founding Fathers intended the Supreme Court to merely discern and apply the original intent of the law. They recall the words of Alexander Hamilton in the *Federalist Papers*, "The judiciary... has no influence over either the sword or the purse... and can take no active resolution whatever. It may truly be said to have neither FORCE nor WILL, but merely judgment." Traditional politicians believe the legislative branch (at both the federal and the state levels) should act as the agent of social change.

The confirmation of Chief Justice John Roberts displayed this polarity of thought. On the first day of Roberts' Senate confirmation hearings, then Democratic Senator Joe Biden framed the issue like this:

> At its core, the Constitution envisions ever-increasing protections for human liberty and dignity for all its citizens and a national government empowered -- empowered -- to

deal with these unanticipated crises.

Judge [Roberts], herein lies, in my view, the crux or the intellectual debate I referred to at the outset: whether we will have an ever-increasing protection for human dignity and human liberty or whether those protections will be diminished, as suggested by many in their reading of the Constitution that says there are no unenumerated rights – theirs is a very narrow reading of the Constitution.[4]

By "unenumerated rights" Biden refers to "rights" that are not specifically defined in the Constitution. In keeping with the postmodern concept of *autonomous freedom*, then Senator Biden believed the "Constitution envisions ever-increasing... human liberty." For the postmodern, to expand liberty is good by definition. Biden believed the crux of the debate was whether or not a Supreme Court Justice would use his or her position to pursue ever-increasing liberties by finding new "unenumerated rights" in the Constitution. Biden rejected the "very narrow" reading of the Constitution that confined a Justice's ruling to the Constitution's original intent. Biden voted against the confirmation of Chief Justice John Roberts on these grounds.

At first Biden's position sounds compassionate. His ideal Supreme Court Justice strove to protect and advance human liberty. Who can argue with such a sentiment? Doesn't the advance of liberty lie at the center of the American dream? However, what happens when the Supreme Court determines one of these "unenumerated rights" is the right of a local government to seize private property to increase its tax revenue as the Court did in *Kelo v. New London*? Recall that Justices Ginsberg and Breyer supported this ruling. Once the Supreme Court is loosed from the bounds of the Constitution's original intent, it becomes an uncontrollable force that threatens, rather than protects, liberty.

Barack Obama voted against the confirmation of John Roberts on similar grounds. In a statement Obama released shortly after the hearings he stated:

The problem I face... is that while adherence to legal precedent and rules of statutory or constitutional construction will dispose of 95 percent of the cases... what matters on the Supreme Court is those 5 percent of cases that are truly difficult. In those cases, adherence to precedent and rules of construction and interpretation will only get you through the 25th mile of the marathon. That last mile can only be determined on the basis of one's deepest values, one's core concerns, one's broader perspectives on how the world works, and *the depth and breadth of one's empathy.*

In those 5 percent of hard cases, the constitutional text will not be directly on point. The language of the statute will not be perfectly clear. Legal process alone will not lead you to a rule of decision. In those circumstances... in those difficult cases, *the critical ingredient is supplied by what is in the judge's heart....*

The problem I had is that when I examined Judge Roberts' record and history of public service, it is my personal estimation that he has far more often used his formidable skills on behalf of the strong in opposition to the weak....

The bottom line is this: I will be voting against John Roberts' nomination. I do so with considerable reticence. I hope that I am wrong... *I hope that he will recognize who the weak are and who the strong are in our society.*[5] (emphasis added)

Obama's statement is remarkable. In taking this position, Obama asserted the Supreme Court should favor one group of Americans over another (namely the weak over the strong), precisely what the rule of law forbids. Had he forgotten the words emblazoned above the entry to the Supreme Court, *"EQUAL JUSTICE UNDER LAW"*? In the most difficult cases, Obama believes a Supreme Court Justice should appeal to empathy and emotion as the basis of their ruling, not the fair and equal application of law. After praising John Roberts at length for his brilliant intellect and commitment to the fair and just application of the law, Obama voted against his confirmation because Roberts would not use his position to help the weak conquer the strong.

In contrast, John Roberts made this observation in his opening statement before the Senate:

> Mr. Chairman, when I worked in the Department of Justice, in the office of the solicitor general, it was my job to argue cases for the United States before the Supreme court.
>
> I always found it very moving to stand before the justices and say, I speak for my country.
>
> But it was after I left the department and began arguing cases against the United States that I fully appreciated the importance of the Supreme Court and our constitutional system.
>
> *Here was the United States, the most powerful entity in the world, aligned against my client. And, yet, all I had to do was convince the court that I was right on the law and the government was wrong and all that power and might would recede in deference to the rule of law. That is a remarkable thing.*
>
> It is what we mean when we say that we are a government of laws and not of men. It is that rule of law that protects the rights and liberties of all Americans. It is the envy of the world. Because without the rule of law, any rights are meaningless.[6] (emphasis added)

Note the enormous difference between the worldviews of John Roberts and Barack Obama. Both Roberts and Obama found it remarkable that in America a common citizen could stand against the power of the United States government. However, where Roberts appealed to a fixed Truth and the rule of law, "*all I had to do was convince the court that I was right on the law,*" Obama appealed to the empathy of the individual Supreme Court Justices.

The profound nature of this difference cannot be overstated. Under John Roberts, *all a citizen had to do was convince the court that he or she was right under the fixed Truth of law.* This assured the ongoing liberty of the common man, regardless of who sat on the Court. Under Barack Obama, liberty for the common man depended on the compassion and empathy of those in power. This is the difference between the American Constitution and the French

Declaration of Human Rights. Under Barack Obama's understanding of a Supreme Court Justice, suddenly our unalienable rights become alienable. Suddenly America finds herself under the rule of Plato's philosopher king. Suddenly liberty depends on the goodwill of government.

When campaigning for the Presidency in July 2007, Obama made this point even more explicit when laying out his criteria for selecting a Supreme Court Justice:

> We need somebody who's got the heart, the empathy, to recognize what it's like to be a young teenage mom. The empathy to understand what it's like to be poor, or African-American, or gay, or disabled, or old. And that's the criteria by which I'm going to be selecting my judges.[7]

However, what happens when the Court has compassion for the State and not the citizen? By redefining the Fifth Amendment words "public use" Justices Ginsberg and Breyer demonstrated empathy for the city of New London, not for Suzette Kelo. Under the ruling of a postmodern Supreme Court, Susette Kelo lost her home.

4) Postmodern Thought Appeals to Foreign Law

Not only do postmodern thinkers set aside the original intent of the Constitution, they look to foreign standards for decision-making, particularly the United Nations and foreign courts. In doing so they subject the United States Constitution to the influence of foreign law. This violates the concept of self-rule that undergirds American freedom.

The profound danger of allowing foreign law to influence interpretation of what our Constitution "should" mean is that foreign law presents Supreme Court Justices a virtual smorgasbord of options from which to choose.

On February 7, 2006, Justice Ginsburg delivered a speech addressing the Supreme Court's use of foreign law. Her introduction voices her support for the United States Supreme Court using foreign law to assist in decision-making:

South Africa's 1996 constitution famously provides in Section 393: "When interpreting the

Bill of Rights, a court... must consider international law; and may consider foreign law" Other modern Constitutions have similar provisions, India's and Spain's, for example. In the United States the question whether and when courts may seek enlightenment from the laws and decisions of other nations has provoked heated debate. I will speak of that controversy in these remarks. At the outset, I should disclose the view I have long held: If U.S. experience and decisions can be instructive to systems that have more recently instituted or invigorated judicial review for constitutionality, so we can learn from others including Canada, South Africa, and most recently the U.K...

The U.S. judicial system will be the poorer, I have urged, if we do not both share our experience with, and learn from, legal systems with values and a commitment to democracy similar to our own.[8]

The profound danger of allowing foreign law to influence interpretation of what our Constitution "should" mean is that nearly any personal preference can find legal support in some other country. The ability to use foreign law presents Supreme Court Justices a virtual smorgasbord of options from which to choose. Loosed from all fixed points of reference, an autonomous Supreme Court would no longer be "beyond comparison, the weakest of the three departments of power."

(Note: The Supreme Court Justices willing to rewrite the Fifth Amendment in the 2005 *Kelo* decision are the same Supreme Court Justices that believe we should look to foreign law. This is deeply troubling.)

5) Postmodern Politicians Find it Difficult to Condemn Reprehensible Behavior Abroad

Chapter Fourteen discussed the postmodern perspective on international confrontation:

Recall the primary tenet of postmodernism—there is no

Universal Truth. "Truth" is what is true for you; "truth" is what is true for me. All sides stand on level ground. The only perspective banned from a postmodern world is one that claims to know the Right. The unforgivable sin? To impose that view on others through military force. To the postmodern mind, this marks the epitome of narrow-minded arrogance. Here we find the source of the Left's anti-military passion....

Postmodern thought litters the political landscape—though, at times, it is difficult to recognize. At first blush it often sounds sophisticated, intellectual, cool, and reasoned. Who could argue with such an evenhanded academic approach? "We must understand all sides without passing judgment." However, because postmodern thought lacks certainty of the good, the right, and the true... in the end, it strips America of the ability to defend liberty.

Recall Mr. Obama's response to Russia's invasions of Georgia in August of 2008. He never distinguished between the aggressor, Russia, and the substantially smaller, invaded U.S. ally and democratic nation Georgia:

I strongly condemn the outbreak of violence in Georgia, and urge an immediate end to armed conflict. Now is the time for Georgia and Russia to show restraint, and to avoid an escalation to full-scale war. Georgia's territorial integrity must be respected. All sides should enter into direct talks on behalf of stability in Georgia, and the United States, the United Nations Security Council, and the international community should fully support a peaceful resolution to this crisis.[9]

A trend took shape in June of 2009 with President Obama's near complete non-involvement during the Green Revolution in Iran. Iran raced toward nuclear weaponry; outside pressures, sanctions, and inspections held little hope of working. Direct military action could lead to a full-scale conflict surpassing the Iraq war in terms of complexity and intensity. The best of all possible outcomes? A Western-friendly regime change fueled from within Iran. With the prospect of a nuclear Iran so imminent, with so few good options to counter, why did President Obama do nothing when the Iranian youth rose to demand freedom? Why was this brief window of opportunity met with nothing but silence from President Obama? His silence became so striking even the protesters in Tehran chanted, "Obama, Obama: You are either with us or with them."[10] Perhaps the incapacitating power of postmodern thought provides the best explanation.

In light of Georgia and Iran, a pattern emerges when one considers President Obama's response to the crisis in Libya. In February of 2011, Colonel Muammar Gaddafi's brutally cracked down on Libyan protesters. Helicopters fired into crowds, militia killed thousands of demonstrators, victims hung from telephone poles, military trucks packed with dead bodies rushed to cover up the carnage, and cash flowed from the dictator in the form of bribes to rat out those leading the protest. In the face of this genocidal evil, Mr. Obama said nothing. Even the Arab League moved to suspend Libya from its membership before the American President spoke.

After a full week of silence Mr. Obama, the last prominent Western leader to address the Libyan crisis, finally issued a statement against violence:

> These actions violate international norms and every standard of common decency. This violence must stop.
>
> The United States also strongly supports the universal rights of the Libyan people. That includes the rights of peaceful assembly, free speech, and the ability of the Libyan people to determine their own destiny. These are human rights. They are not negotiable. They must be respected in every country. And they cannot be denied through violence or suppression.
>
> In a volatile situation like this one, it is imperative that the nations and peoples of the world speak with one voice, and that has been our focus. Yesterday a unanimous U.N. Security

301

Council sent a clear message that it condemns the violence in Libya, supports accountability for the perpetrators, and stands with the Libyan people....

I've also asked Secretary Clinton to travel to Geneva on Monday, where a number of foreign ministers will convene for a session of the Human Rights Council.[11]

The fact the President's first prepared public address only condemned "violence" was noteworthy. This was precisely the language he used two and a half years earlier when Russia invaded Georgia. Nowhere in the entire address entire did Mr. Obama mention Gaddafi, not even once. Nor did the he mention Gaddafi ordered the 1988 bombing of Pan Am Flight 103 that killed 189 Americans. As with Georgia, the toughest action the leader of the free world offered was an appeal to the United Nations Human Rights Council—the same Human Rights Council Libya chaired in 2003.

The President attributed his moderate tone to the fact diplomats in Tripoli warned that "certain kinds of messaging from the American government could endanger the security of American citizens."[12] Many in the media initially applauded the President's delay as a sign of his discretion. However, giving in to a hostage crisis—when there were no hostages—signaled to terrorists around the world that America was now the weak horse. In an essay entitled "Barack Obama's Moral Concession to Evil," Peter Wehner framed the political implications like this:

> On a more fundamental level, what the Obama administration did was create quite a dangerous precedent. It has now signaled to the most malevolent regimes in the world that the way to delay (or perhaps even avoid) American condemnation, let alone American action, is to threaten the lives of American citizens. The message sent to, and surely the message received by, despots around the world is this: If you want to neuter America, threaten to harm its citizens. Mr. Obama will bend like red-hot steel pulled from a furnace.
>
> There were, of course, other options available to the

president, including informing Mr. Qaddafi through the appropriate channels that a terrible fate would await him and his pack of jackals if a single American was harmed. The president did very nearly the opposite. He showed weakness, irresolution, fear. I wonder if people have focused on just how troubling this action, and the mindset it manifests, really is....

For those who were disturbed by President Obama's diffidence in the face of Qaddafi's wickedness, it's worse than you think. The ramifications of Mr. Obama's actions will outlive whatever happens in Tripoli.[13]

One month after the Libyan rebellion began British Prime Minister David Cameron had announced plans for a no-fly zone. French President Nicolas Sarkozy had established diplomatic ties with the Libyan opposition. The Arab League had formally called for Western military intervention in the form of a no-fly zone. Yet, Mr. Obama remained disengaged—even as analysts warned of a possible rebel defeat. In an interview with the *Gaurdian* Mustafa Gheriani, a spokesman for the rebel forces in Benghazi, revealed the consequences of continued disengagement. The report read in part:

A large French flag hangs on the front of the courthouse used as the revolutionary council's headquarters after Paris recognized the rebel leadership, and the tricolour is often seen on the streets of Benghazi. But Libyans are also increasingly vocal in their criticism of Washington in particular for what is seen as a failure to back up rhetoric against the regime.

However, Gheriani said that if the west failed to offer practical help to the revolutionaries to free themselves from Gaddafi's rule it risked frustrated Libyans turning to religious extremists.

The west is missing the point. The revolution was started because people were feeling despair from poverty, from oppression. Their last hope was freedom. If the west takes too long—where people say it's too little, too late—then people become a target for extremists who say the west doesn't care about them,' he said.

'Most people in this country are moderates and extremists have not been able to penetrate them. But if they get to the point of disillusionment with the west there will be no going back.'[14]

While postmodern thinkers sound sophisticated, levelheaded, and intellectual, in the end, postmodern thought strips America of her ability to defend freedom. *If we believe all sides stand on equal ground, if we no longer see ourselves as the defenders of the truly good and right, we lose our capacity to defend the liberties we so dearly love.* The danger of being immersed in a culture of absolute moral neutrality is that we never fully grasp the nature of evil. Nor do we possess the resolve needed to remain free.

The most disturbing aspect of this story emerged as this book went to press. Desperate to avoid ownership of another war, President Obama referred to his sustained missile attack on a foreign country, not as a war, but as a "kinetic military action." He then announced NATO would rapidly assume control of the operation. Nothing could express postmodern thought more clearly.

Supporting the Libyan rebels with military intervention then rapidly turning control of the operation over to NATO appeared to be a brilliant political move. It let President Obama appear decisive even as he distanced himself from the consequences of his decision. Should the effort go badly, NATO would shoulder the blame.

Yet, delegating the duties of Commander-and-Chief to a multinational body proves profoundly disconcerting, if not unconstitutional. Giving foreign leaders command authority over American servicemen and servicewomen not only blurs the chain-of-command, it sets a profoundly dangerous precedent—it places America's ability to defend herself under foreign control.

(Note: This discussion does not address the intensely complex issues surrounding military engagement in multiple Muslim countries. Nor does it suggest such a plan. The central concern here is that postmodern thought weakens America's ability to defend herself and hamstrings her capacity to fight for freedom and liberty around the world.)

6) Postmodern Thought Endorses the Concept of Global Governnce

Recall the fundamental tenet of postmodern thought—no one can claim to know Truth; each point of view is equally valid. According to the postmodern worldview every nation, metaphorically speaking, sits at King Arthur's roundtable; every country has an equal voice. Under a postmodern worldview the United States has no claim to the moral high ground. No institution embodies this worldview better than the United Nations. Three brief examples reveal how postmodern politicians can gradually place America under the authority of the United Nations and "global governance."

— In his book *Winning the Future* Newt Gingrich describes the willingness of some elected officials to subject the American voter to U.N. authority:

> In July 2004, about a dozen House [of Representatives] members wrote a letter to United Nations Secretary General Kofi Annan asking him to certify the 2004 presidential election. When an amendment was offered to block any federal official involving the U.N. in the American elections, the Democrats voted 160 to 33 in favor of allowing the U.N. to be called into an American election. The Republicans voted 210 to 0 against allowing the United Nations to interfere.[15]

This vote is astounding. At stake is nothing less than the autonomy of American elections—the ability of *we the people* to independently choose our leadership. Given the Unites Nation's overt anti-American bias, this is of great concern. Remarkably, 83% of Democratic congressional leaders (160 of 193 votes cast) wished to subject American elections to the authority of the United Nations. In stark contrast, 100% of Republican congressional leaders believed the American voter held final authority. Not all Democrats are postmodern and not all Republicans hold a traditional worldview. However,

The danger of being immersed in a culture of absolute moral neutrality is that we never fully grasp the nature of evil. Nor do we possess the resolve to remain free.

this vote demonstrates a marked polarity of worldviews between the leadership of the two parties.

— When still in the Senate, Barack Obama (cosponsored by Joe Biden and 29 others, see Appendix I) introduced Senate Bill S. 2433 titled the *Global Poverty Act of 2007*. The bill used language that appeals to the best of American values—reducing global poverty. However, if passed, this bill would obligate the American taxpayer to give the United Nations an estimated 65 billion additional dollars each year.[16]

Reducing global poverty is undoubtedly a worthy goal. However, does funneling this staggering sum of money through an organization characterized by corruption and inefficiency best achieve this goal? Is this the most effective use of taxpayer dollars and does it improve American goodwill overseas, or will some of this money actually be used against America's own interests? More than any other nation on Earth, Americans already reach out to the poorest of the poor on a global scale, but they do so through private efforts. Not only are privately donated dollars used more efficiently, but people in third world countries see the generosity of the American people firsthand, rather than placing their trust in the United Nations.

Once the American taxpayer becomes responsible for eliminating global poverty, the concept of America as an autonomous, self-governing nation disappears. One is reminded of Barack Obama's claim to be a "citizen of the world" while in Germany during the summer of 2008. He went on to say to the tens-of-thousands of German citizens, "People of Berlin, people of the world, this is our moment. This is our time."[17] These words seem more befitting of a World Supreme Leader, not the next President of the United States.

— New to political American political discourse is the concept of "global governance" as a viable reality. The idea gained prominence following the Kyoto Protocol discussions. On November 20, 2000 French President Jacques Chirac noted:

> For the first time, humanity is instituting a genuine instrument of global governance. From the very earliest age, we should make environmental awareness a major theme

of education and a major theme of political debate, until respect for the environment comes to be as fundamental as safeguarding our rights and freedoms. By acting together, by building this unprecedented instrument, the first component of an authentic global governance, we are working for dialogue and peace.[18]

That a foreign leader seeks to place the United States under a global power is not particularly noteworthy. However, when this language comes from a former American Vice-president, Americans have reason for concern. On July 7, 2009 former Vice-president Al Gore applauded global governance in a speech in London. Gore said:

I bring you good news from the United States. Within one month of taking office President Obama secured 80 billion dollars U.S. for renewable energy and green infrastructure. Then just two weeks ago, the House of Representatives passed the Waxman-Markey bill, which for all of its flaws does put a price on carbon and is very much a step in the right direction....

But it is the awareness itself that will drive the change. And one of the ways it will drive the change is through global governance and global agreements.[19]

The *autonomous freedom* promised by postmodern thought initially sounded so sweet. But in the end, *we the people* risk losing our independence. Every two years we go to the polls. Here, and in the American classroom, we must defend our freedom.

Time to Act

Mahatma Gandhi once said, "If I seem to take part in politics, it is only because politics encircles us today like the coil of a snake from which one cannot get out, no matter how much one tries. I wish therefore to wrestle with the snake." Like Gandhi, we must wrestle the snake.

In this battle of worldviews, America is rapidly losing its moral compass, unable to differentiate good from evil. Infanticide hovers at our doorstep. Culture robs children of both meaning and innocence. Postmodern thought strips our universities of the capacity to discriminate between freedom and tyranny. Political leaders explicitly violate the rule of law without consequence. Local governments seize private property for financial gain. The most powerful nation on earth finds itself impotent in the face of genocide, and America now contemplates surrendering its autonomy to a world body. Yet, this insanity does not form in a vacuum; it is the logical conclusion of America's choice to follow the road of postmodern thought.

Postmodern thought floods our culture largely because those who hold traditional values engaged the debate on the wrong ground. Traditional Americans often argue in the present using thought forms of the past, and their voices go unheard. Contemporary culture no longer understands their language. As the universal acceptance of thesis/antithesis and the principal of non-contradiction fade into forgotten history, classical logic no longer affects the postmodern mind.

Now, truth is what is "true" for me. Using the thought form of thesis/antithesis, the conservative now futilely argues against a mindset that has no fixed point of reference… yet, this is not quite true. In reality, the conservative argues against a thought form that maintains the only absolute is that *no one else* can claim an absolute. America's cultural divide is fundamentally not about *what we think, but how.*

Before our eyes, Reason is being reshaped into non-Reason as postmodern thought destroys the foundation that makes true liberty possible. When the basis of liberty is removed, a new kind of freedom will emerge that knows no bounds—a freedom *from* the rule of law that will destroy the liberty of the common man. It has been said there are laws that enslave men's souls and there are laws that set men free. As we stand at the crossroads of culture, which will it be?

Our nation faces a clear choice between two alternative futures. One returns to the wisdom of the Founding Fathers where the concepts of a fixed Truth and the "laws of nature and nature's God" secure true freedom for the common man. The other marches down the road of historicism following the doctrine of inexorable progress; change is good no matter where that change leads.

Though America now travels the road of postmodern thought and autonomous freedom, hope remains if *we the people* awaken and find the courage to respond to the call of history once again. We must restore our courts, our classrooms, and our political leadership. We must remember the wisdom of our Founding Fathers, for in their thinking we find the foundations of a true and lasting liberty.

The trumpet of Truth now summons us to engage in the eternal fight for human freedom. A new force seeks to consume America, one that cannot be fought with sword or rifle but only with insight into its nature. As Sun-tsu warns, we must know our enemy; we must understand the consuming power of postmodern thought and declare with John F. Kennedy:

> Let the word go forth from this time and place, to friend and foe alike, that the torch has been passed to a new generation of Americans—born in this century, tempered by war, disciplined by a hard and bitter peace, proud of our ancient heritage—and unwilling to witness or permit the slow undoing of those human rights to which this nation has always been committed, and to which we are committed today at home and around the world.
>
> Let every nation know, whether it wishes us well or ill, that we shall pay any price, bear any burden, meet any hardship, support any friend, oppose any foe to assure the survival and success of liberty.[20]

A cultural chasm yawns before America—the direct result of a change in the concept of Truth. Let us remember our heritage, return to the foundations that made our country the greatest nation on earth, and pray for the healing of this great nation. Let us recapture the vision of President Reagan so America may once again glisten as a shining city on a hill. Let us restore the soul of our beloved country so she can once again stand as a beacon of hope to a world in need. We can and we will, because in the end, freedom still runs red through our veins.

Notes

1   C. S. Lewis, *The Abolition of Man*, (New York: Simon & Schuster, 1996), p. 37.

2   Michael Barone, "White House puts UAW ahead of property rights," *The Washington Examiner*, May 5, 2009. http://washingtonexaminer.com/politics/2009/05/white-house-puts-uaw-ahead-property-rights

3   Patient Protection and Affordable Care Act, Section 3007, Value-Based Payment Modifier Under the Physician Fee Schedule, January 5, 2010, pp. 274.

4   Joe Biden, Transcript: Day One of the Roberts Hearings, September 13, 2005.

5   Barack Obama, Remarks of Senator Barack Obama on the Confirmation of Judge John Roberts, September 22, 2005.

6   John Roberts, Opening Statement in the Senate Confirmation Hearings, September 12, 2005.

7   Barack Obama, "Barack Obama and the Supreme Court," Fox News, October 22, 2008. http://www.foxnews.com/story/0,2933,443644,00.html

8   Ruth Bader Ginsburg, Supreme Court Associate Justice, *A Decent Respect to the Opinions of [Human]kind, The Value of a Comparative Perspective in Constitutional Adjudication*, February 7, 2006.

9   Statement from Barack Obama on the Grave Situation in Georgia, August 8, 2008, www.barackobama.com

10   Charles Krauthammer, "Protesters beg for U.S. help, but Obama waits and waits," The Register Guard, March 7, 2011.

11   President Obama, President Obama Speak on the Turmoil in Libya: 'This Violence Must Stop'", The White House Blog, February 23, 2011. http://www.whitehouse.gov/blog/2011/02/23/president-obama-speaks-turmoil-libya-violence-must-stop

12   Scott Wilson, "White House caution in response to Gaddafi's actions was guided by fears for the safety of Americans in Libya," *Washington Post*, February 27, 2011. http://www.washingtonpost.com/wp-dyn/content/article/2011/02/26/AR2011022604003.html

13   Peter Wehner, "Barack Obama's Moral Concession to Evil," Commentary Magazine, February 28, 2011. http://www.commentarymagazine.com/2011/02/28/barack-obama's-moral-concession-to-evil/

14   Chris McGreal, "Libyan rebels urge west to assassinate Gaddafi as his forces near Benghazi," *Guardian.co.uk*, March 14, 2011. http://www.guardian.co.uk/world/2011/mar/14/libyan-rebel-leaders-gaddafi-benghazi

15   Newt Gingrich, *Winning the Future*, (Washington, DC: Regnery Publishing, 2005), p. 71.

16   Cliff Kincaid, "Obama's Global Tax Proposal Up for Senate Vote," Accuracy in Media, February 12, 2008. http://www.aim.org/aim-column/obamas-global-tax-

proposal-up-for-senate-vote/
17   Barack Obama, Berlin speech, July 27, 2008.
18   Jacques Chirac, Speech at The Haague, November 20, 2000. http://www.
     climatedepot.com/a/1893/Gore-US-Climate-Bill-Will-Help-Bring-About-Global-
     Governance
19   Al Gore, "Smith School Forum on Enterprise and the Environment," London,
     July 7, 2009.
20   John F. Kennedy, *Inaugural Address*, 20 January 1961.

SPONSOR AND CO-SPONSORS FOR BILL S. 2433

How can voters identify a postmodern politician? This is a list of Senators willing to transfer hundreds of billions of American dollars to the United Nations. Subjecting America to the authority of the United Nations is a hallmark of the postmodern politician.

This bill places the U.S. taxpayer under the control of foreign world leaders and needlessly empowers an institution that often seeks to undermine America. While reducing global poverty is a noble goal, America does not have to surrender authority to the United Nations to pursue it.

Sponsor

Sen. Barack Obama

Democratic Co-Sponsors

1. Sen. Joseph Biden [D-DE]
2. Sen. Jeff Bingaman [D-NM]
3. Sen. Barbara Boxer [D-CA]
4. Sen. Sherrod Brown [D-OH]
5. Sen. Maria Cantwell [D-CA]
6. Sen. Benjamin Cardin [D-MD]
7. Sen. Robert Casey [D-PA]

8. Sen. Hillary Clinton [D-NY]

9. Sen. Christopher Dodd [D-CT]

10. Sen. Richard Durbin [D-IL]

11. Sen. Russell Feingold [D-WI]

12. Sen. Dianne Feinstein [D-CA]

13. Sen. Tom Harkin [D-IA]

14. Sen. Tim Johnson [D-SD]

15. Sen. John Kerry [D-MA]

16. Sen. Amy Klobuchar [D-MN]

17. Sen. Herbert Kohl [D-WI]

18. Sen. Frank Lautenberg [D-NJ]

19. Sen. Robert Menendez [D-NJ]

20. Sen. Barbara Mikulski [D-MD]

21. Sen. Patty Murray [D-WA]

22. Sen. Charles Schumer [D-MD]

23. Sen. Debbie Ann Stabenow [D-MI]

24. Sen. Jim Webb [D-VA]

25. Sen. Ron Wyden [D-OR]

Republican Co-Sponsors

1. Sen. Susan Collins [R-ME]

2. Sen. Charles Hagel [R-NE]

3. Sen. Richard Lugar [R-IN]

4. Sen. Gordon Smith [R-OR]

5. Sen. Olympia Snow [R-ME]

Acknowledgements

Over the years, scores of people wished me well in this effort and I remain thankful for their support. However, I owe two individuals a special debt of gratitude. Their gifts of time and encouragement gave me strength to persevere in an undertaking so massive it required fifteen years to complete.

First, I want to thank my mother. She deserves consideration for sainthood for the countless hours she listened to me struggle to discern how men such as Plato, Aristotle, Descartes, and Nietzsche influenced contemporary thought and culture. Only a mother would show endless patience for such an obscure subject. Without her support and listening ear this book would have never reached completion. I will remain forever grateful for her loving footprints that canvass the path of my life.

Second, I must thank Marylane Wade Koch. With patient devotion, Marylane not only served as my editor, she became a mentor, coach, confidant, and friend. Marylane adopted me when I was little more than a novice writer. However, even then she believed I wrote with passion and purpose. Over a period of several years she skillfully guided me through repeated rewritings of the manuscript. With each successive revision, the foundations of the American culture war emerged with increasing clarity. In the end, we transformed what resembled a doctoral thesis into a story that engages the heartfelt passions of the American patriot.

Finally, I thank God for His continued guidance and for the many people He brought into my life who gave me their friendship, love, and support in this project.

About the Author

Dr. C. L. Gray is a nationally recognized writer, speaker, and board certified physician practicing hospital-based medicine in western North Carolina. In 2006 he founded Physicians for Reform, a non-profit organization dedicated to preserving patient-centered healthcare. The Battle for America's Soul resulted from a decade spent in research and analysis of the history and philosophy of medical ethics. This book presents findings that link America's present cultural divide with the practice of Post-Hippocratic medicine.

As one of the nation's leading patient advocates, Dr. Gray has written multiple op-eds for publications such as *The Washington Times, Investors Business Daily, The Washington Examiner*, and *The Hill*. With some 400,000 readers, Gray's *Why Doctors are Leaving Medicare* became one of the most frequently read opinion pieces posted by FOX News.

Gray's work has taken him to Washington and Raleigh, NC where *Physicians for Reform* works to help craft solutions to save Medicare and Medicaid from financial collapse. Physicians recently underwent the longest interruption of payments in Medicare's history. This places seniors at risk as doctors abandon Medicare in record numbers. These and other devastating dilemmas can only be solved through patient-centered, fiscally responsible reforms such as outlined by *Physicians for Reform*.

CPSIA information can be obtained at www.ICGtesting.com
Printed in the USA
BVOW041127030912

299440BV00008B/150/P